HISTORY TAKING

FOR MEDICAL FINALS

Joshua Michaels

MBBS, BSc Clinical Sciences (cardiovascular medicine) Intercalation

Foundation Year 1 Doctor, Leeds Teaching Hospitals NHS Trust

Scion

© Scion Publishing Limited, 2018

ISBN 9781911510222

First published 2018

A CIP catalogue record for this book is available from the British Library.

Scion Publishing Limited

The Old Hayloft, Vantage Business Park, Bloxham Road, Banbury OX16 9UX, UK
www.scionpublishing.com

Important Note from the Publisher

The information contained within this book was obtained by Scion Publishing Ltd from sources believed by us to be reliable. However, while every effort has been made to ensure its accuracy, no responsibility for loss or injury whatsoever occasioned to any person acting or refraining from action as a result of information contained herein can be accepted by the authors or publishers.

Readers are reminded that medicine is a constantly evolving science and while the authors and publishers have ensured that all dosages, applications and practices are based on current indications, there may be specific practices which differ between communities. You should always follow the guidelines laid down by the manufacturers of specific products and the relevant authorities in the country in which you are practising.

Although every effort has been made to ensure that all owners of copyright material have been acknowledged in this publication, we would be pleased to acknowledge in subsequent reprints or editions any omissions brought to our attention.

Registered names, trademarks, etc. used in this book, even when not marked as such, are not to be considered unprotected by law.

Typeset by Phoenix Photosetting Ltd, Chatham, UK
Printed in the UK

Contents

Preface   vii
About the author   viii
Acknowledgments   viii
Abbreviations   ix

Introduction   1

1   Psychiatry   3
1.1   Anxiety   5
1.2   Depression   10
1.3   Mania   14
1.4   Psychosis   18

2   Musculoskeletal   21
2.1   Arthritis   23
2.2   Back pain   28
2.3   Head trauma   32

3   Oncology   35
3.1   Breast cancer   37
3.2   Haematological cancer   40

4   Respiratory   43
4.1   Shortness of breath   45
4.2   Cough   51

5   Cardiovascular   55
5.1   Chest pain (acute)   57
5.2   Chest pain (chronic)   62
5.3   Peripheral vascular disease   65
5.4   Valvular history   69
5.5   Arrhythmias   72

6	**Neurology**	**75**
6.1	Headache	77
6.2	Vertigo	81
6.3	Weakness	83
6.4	Neuropathy	88
6.5	Epilepsy	90
6.6	Parkinson's disease	92
6.7	Eye	94
7	**Gastrointestinal**	**97**
7.1	Liver	99
7.2	GI bleed	102
7.3	Abdominal pain	105
7.4	Change in bowel habit	109
7.5	Dysphagia	112
8	**Women's health**	**115**
8.1	Infertility	117
8.2	Pregnancy	120
8.3	PV bleed	123
8.4	Pelvic pain	126
8.5	Amenorrhoea	128
9	**Endocrine**	**131**
9.1	Thyroid	133
9.2	Diabetes	136
10	**Urology/renal**	**141**
10.1	Urology	143
10.2	Renal history	145
10.3	Example renal consultation	148
11	**Paediatrics**	**151**
11.1	General paediatric protocol	153

Preface

The purpose of this book is to provide a succinct review of how to take a history to the standard expected of a final year medical student. It is easily laid out to facilitate your learning process, and is very clear, focused and thorough. Superfluous information, which would otherwise amount to a large and inaccessible piece of text, has been removed.

The book focuses on taking a history from various presenting complaints, accommodating both acute and chronic situations. I will take you through each 'step' of the history, covering symptomatic red flags and pertinent information which it is essential you discover. Specifically during a clinical exam, which is a high pressured and intense situation, the purpose of the clinical history is to provide the examiner with an insight into your thought process. The way to achieve that, very simply, is to ask the 'right' questions, demonstrating you are SAFE and competent.

My personal philosophy underlying any clinical exam is to "read the rule book and play the game". This book is the rule book. You simply have to play and execute. A clinical exam is a theatre performance. The clinical setting is your stage, the patient your fellow actor and the examiner your audience. You simply need to learn your lines. This book will provide you with the tools to put on the performance necessary to acquire those crucial marks.

Good luck and happy playing!

Joshua Michaels
January 2018

Introduction

You will frequently be told about adhering to the patient's agenda. This basically means that you must allow the patient to dictate the consultation according to their needs. In terms of a 'real-life' situation this is wholly relevant, especially in a GP setting where the patient is likely to have rehearsed their opening statement numerous times. Furthermore, the 'Golden Minute', which is allowing the patient to speak for approximately a minute before interception, is significant. If you allow this to happen, it is likely that a large majority of the information you would otherwise have had to accrue will be covered.

Both these principles need to be adhered to; however, this is *your* exam. *You* must take control of the history. You have a limited amount of time to demonstrate to your examiner that you are SAFE. To do this, you need to ask the 'right' questions. This is why having a standard structure and a set number of questions for each presenting complaint acts as an absolute failsafe. I have purposely ensured that you screen for all **RED FLAGS** as well as cover all necessary aspects of the history for each presenting complaint. Furthermore, please note that repetition and consistency lead to success. By its very nature this book should be studied like a script; it is thus intentionally repetitive.

Taking control of the history, which basically means asserting your own agenda, directly contradicts the need to allow the patient to do the same. This can be done subtly, however. Listening is important, and what I strongly advise is using each statement from the patient to word your next question. It demonstrates you have listened AND followed on from what *they* have said. It creates the illusion of adhering to their agenda when you are subtly imposing your own by using *their* words to form *your* questions.

1.1 Anxiety

Summary of steps required

1. Take an adequate history of the presenting complaint
2. Time period
3. Establish a history of these episodes
4. Directly address their concerns
5. Assess their premorbid personality
6. Identify triggers
7. Identify coping mechanisms
8. Assess the impact on their mood/life, etc.

Hint alert

Anxiety can manifest in many ways. The patient could be suffering from one of the following:

- *Generalized anxiety disorder (GAD)*
- *Anxiety attacks*
- *Panic attacks*
- *Specific phobias*
- *Obsessive–compulsive disorder (OCD)*
- *Agoraphobia*
- *Post-traumatic stress disorder (PTSD)*
- *Acute stress reaction*
- *Grief reaction*

Your aim is to find out which type of anxiety the patient is suffering from. To achieve your aim, you must ask the right questions. The structure of your history and the questions you should ask are given below.

Step 1   Take an adequate history of the presenting complaint

Your patient could present with a multitude of non-specific, vague symptoms such as palpitations, sweating, breathlessness, headaches, over-heating and so forth. Your aim during *Step 1* is to simply acquire an understanding of the situation. The following questions will facilitate that process:

- *"What symptoms/feelings do you start to experience?"*
- *"When did these symptoms/feelings start to occur?"*
- *"How frequently do they occur?"*
- *"When these symptoms/feelings start to develop, how long do they affect you for?"*
- *"Are there any particular situations which seem to correlate with the emergence of these symptoms/feelings?"*

hyperventilation and sweating. Furthermore, *Step 1* is purposely brief as the remaining aspects of the history will cover additional aspects in adequate depth.

Step 2   Time period

- *"How long has this been happening for?"*

Technique alert

Every question you ask has a purpose. Establishing the time period is crucial, and will facilitate your fundamental diagnosis. Has this been for 2–3 days, raising suspicion of an *acute stress reaction*, or 3–4 weeks, raising suspicions for *GAD*? There must always be a purpose behind each question you ask.

Step 3   Establish a history of these episodes

- *"Have you had thoughts/feelings/episodes like this in the past?"*

Step 4   Directly address their concerns

- *"What are your main concerns?"*

Technique alert

This follows on nicely from the previous two questions. If this has been happening for 3–4 weeks and the patient has not experienced an episode like this in the past (information you've gathered from *Steps 2* and *3*), the patient may be scared and unsure. If it is a specific phobia – for example, public speaking – and they have recently acquired a new job which involves running meetings or presenting business ideas, they will understandably be concerned about their ability to perform optimally, and, by default, the risk of losing their job. Obtaining this information, which is frequently missed, helps build patient rapport and ticks boxes from an examiner's perspective.

1.2 Depression

Summary of steps required

1. Take an adequate history of the presenting complaint
2. Time period
3. Establish a history of these episodes
4. Directly address their concerns
5. Assess their premorbid personality
6. Identify triggers
7. Identify coping mechanisms
8. Assess the impact on their mood/life, etc.

Hint alert

Depression can manifest in many ways. The patient could be suffering from one of the following:

- *Overt, basic depression (know the diagnostic criteria)*
- *Bipolar affective disorder*
- *Seasonal affective disorder*
- *Psychotic depression (the psychosis can be picked up in the mental state examination)*
- *Postnatal depression*
- *Atypical presentation of depression (e.g. memory loss in the elderly)*
- *Normal sadness*

It is important to note that the presentation of depression can vary considerably. The patient may present with tiredness, memory loss, poor sleeping pattern, etc. Although quite confusing in that it may not be a simple presentation of 'low mood', the presentation will still be a key symptom of *depression*.

Hint alert: diagnostic criteria for depression

Depression is defined as being the presence of at least four of the symptoms listed below, two of which must be of the key three symptoms (down, lack energy, anhedonia), for at least two weeks.

DEPRESSION
Down
Energy (lack of)
Pleasure (lack of – anhedonia)
Retardation (psychomotor)
Energy
Sleep
Suicide
I'm a failure
Only me to blame
No concentration

Libido is also important (the first symptom to come and go).

Step 1   **Take an adequate history of the presenting complaint**

There will likely be a story, e.g. *"I have recently separated from my husband."*

Utilize the history to feed your questioning so you can subtly screen for the symptoms of **'DEPRESSION'**.

It may also be necessary to screen for the following organic, physical causes as mentioned above, especially if it is a vague presentation such as *'tiredness'*.
- Underlying malignancy – *"Have you experienced any recent weight loss?"*
- Hyper-/hypothyroidism (recent development of a tremor, palpitations, sweating, weight fluctuations, heat (in)tolerance, visual disturbances, neck swelling, muscle stiffness, change in bowel habit and/or menstruation pattern)
- Hyper-/hypoparathyroidism
- Diabetes
- Anaemia (may be part of a haematological condition causing pancytopenia so query any recent bleeding/ bruising or infection/fever).

Step 2   Time period

- *"How long has this been happening for?"*

Step 3   Establish a history of these episodes

- *"Have you had thoughts/feelings/episodes like this in the past?"*

Step 4   Directly address their concerns

- *"What are your main concerns?"*

Step 5   Assess their premorbid personality

- *"You mentioned this has been going on for 3 months now, and you've never experienced thoughts and feelings like this in the past. Bearing that in mind, if you take me back to before this particular episode started to happen, how would you describe your personality?*
- *"How would others describe your personality?"*

Step 6   Identify triggers

- *"The person you have just described seems very different to the one sitting in front of me today* [again, use the information you've acquired from previous questions to word your next question]*; can you think of any reason as to why you are currently experiencing these thoughts and feelings?"*
- *"Can you think of any triggers?"*

Step 7   Identify coping mechanisms

"Many people experiencing these thoughts and feelings can develop coping strategies; have you developed any coping strategies?"

It is likely they will ask: *"What do you mean?"*

Your reply might be: *"Well, some people can develop positive coping strategies such as ..."*

Offer a few suggestions such as talking to family members and friends. You are subtly establishing the extent of their support network. If they have a limited support network, that could mean they're isolated, which is concerning.

"Furthermore, some people develop negative coping strategies such as..." Again, detail some of these and use the opportunity to screen for recreational medication and alcohol use.

Step 8   **Assess the impact on their mood/life, etc.**

Make sure you ask whether there have been times when their mood has been the opposite, i.e. when they have experienced elation and boundless energy. You are screening for bipolar.

Remember to ask
• Past medical history
• Past psychiatric history
• Past surgical history
• Are you known to the police?
• Drug history and allergies
• Family history
• Social history

> **Technique alert**
>
> Here, you are screening for family members and friends. If they haven't, why not? Do they feel in danger? What do they think would happen if they told someone? Have they not actually got any family/friends to tell? If not, then they're isolated, which is worrying.

Step 5   Time period

- *"When did you first become aware you had this extraordinary ability?"*

If this was relatively recently (e.g. over a fortnight), it raises suspicion of an acute trigger such as recreational medication use.

Step 6   Establish a history of these episodes

- *"Have you had thoughts/feelings/episodes like this in the past?"*

Step 7   Assess their premorbid personality

- *"You mentioned this has been going on for three months now, and you've never experienced thoughts and feelings like this in the past. Bearing that in mind, if you take me back to before this particular episode started to happen, how would you describe your personality?"*
- *"How would others describe your personality?"*

Step 8   Identify triggers

- *"The person you have just described seems very different to the one sitting in front of me today* [again, using the information you've acquired from previous questions to word your next question]*; can you think of any reason why you are currently experiencing these thoughts and feelings?"*
- *"Can you think of any triggers?"*
- *"Furthermore, have you recently been taking recreational medication and/or drinking alcohol in excess?"*

Technique alert

It is strongly advised that you specifically ask about alcohol and recreational drug use as part of your 'triggers' screen (see also *Step 5*). One of the reasons for this is because there is not a 'coping mechanisms' step. This is due to the fact that people with mania lack insight and thus do not believe they need to 'cope'.

Step 9   Assess the impact on their mood/life, etc.

Make sure you ask whether there have been times when their mood has been the opposite, i.e. pervasive low mood and lack of energy. You are screening for bipolar.

Remember to ask

- Past medical history
- Past psychiatric history
- Past surgical history
- Are you known to the police?
- Drug history and allergies
- Family history
- Social history

1.4 Psychosis

Summary of steps required

1. Take an adequate history of the presenting complaint
2. Time period
3. Establish a history of these episodes
4. Directly address their concerns
5. Assess the impact on their mood/life, etc.
6. Assess their premorbid personality
7. Identify triggers
8. Identify coping mechanisms

Hint alert

Psychosis is a syndrome, not a diagnosis. The patient may be suffering from one of the following:

- *Schizophrenia* (which subtype?)
- *Schizoaffective disorder*
- *Bipolar affective disorder*
- *Drug-induced psychosis*
- *Psychotic depression*
- *Delusional disorder*
- *Brief psychotic episode*

Diagnostic criteria for schizophrenia
The presence of at least one of Kurt Schneider's First-Rank Symptoms or persistent delusion for at least 1 month with no current drug withdrawal/intoxication, overt brain disease or prominent affective symptoms.

Kurt Schneider's First-Rank Symptoms
- *Third person auditory hallucinations*
- *Thought echo*
- *Thought insertion, withdrawal, broadcast*
- *Passivity*
- *Delusional perception*

Step 1   **Take an adequate history of the presenting complaint**

Screen for Kurt Schneider's First-Rank Symptoms by utilizing the history accordingly.

A typical example of how to screen for your first-rank symptoms (these have to be asked in the relevant context of your patient's presentation):
- *"Do you feel like your thoughts can be manipulated?"*
- *"Do you feel like your feelings and your emotions can be controlled?"*
- *"Can you hear people talking when others cannot?"*
- *"Do you ever see or hear things that you feel are giving a message that is specific to you?"*

Step 2   **Time period**

- *"How long has this been happening for?"*

Step 3   **Establish a history of these episodes**

- *"Have you had thoughts/feelings like this in the past?"*

Step 4   **Directly address their concerns**

- *"What are your main concerns?"*

Step 5   **Assess the impact on their mood/life, etc.**

- *"What impact is this having on your mood?"*

Screen for depressive symptoms.

Step 6   **Assess their premorbid personality**

- *"You mentioned this has been going on for 3 months now, and you've never experienced thoughts and feelings like this in the past. Bearing that in mind, if you take me back to before this particular episode started to happen, how would you describe your personality?"*
- *"How would others describe your personality?"*

Step 7   Identify triggers

- *"The person you have just described seems very different to the one sitting in front of me today* [again, using the information you've acquired from previous questions to word your next question]*; can you think of any reason why you are currently experiencing these thoughts and feelings?"*
- *"Can you think of any triggers?"*

Step 8   Identify coping mechanisms

"Many people experiencing these thoughts and feelings can develop coping strategies; have you developed any coping strategies?"

It is likely they will ask: *"What do you mean?"*

Your reply might be: *"Well, some people can develop positive coping strategies such as..."*

Offer a few suggestions such as talking to family members and friends. You are subtly establishing the extent of their support network. If they have a limited support network, that could mean they're isolated, which is concerning.

"Furthermore, some people develop negative coping strategies such as..." Again, offer some examples and use the opportunity to screen for recreational medication and alcohol use.

Remember to ask

- Past medical history
- Past psychiatric history
- Past surgical history
- Are you known to the police?
- Drug history and allergies
- Family history
- Social history

Chapter 2

Musculoskeletal

Scenarios presented

2.1   Arthritis 23

2.2   Back pain 28

2.3   Head trauma 32

Possible scenarios to practise

Chronic pain

Frozen shoulder

Tennis elbow

Your systemic screen includes brief questions to gauge how unwell the patient is. Do not ask questions for each physiological system – this is an arbitrary and time-wasting technique.

Step 7   Create a differential

"There are lots of things that may be responsible for causing joint pain/stiffness, so I'm going to ask a few very important screening questions."

Then ask the following:
- *"When the joint pain initially started, did you develop any ulcers in your mouth?"* (Behçet's disease)
- *"Have you noticed any skin rashes/lesions, specifically on your elbows or knees?"* (psoriatic arthritis)
- *"When you developed the joint pain, did you have a corresponding change in bowel habit or any urinary symptoms?"* (reactive arthritis)
- *"This is a sensitive question but an important one – when you initially developed the joint problem, had you recently had any unprotected sexual intercourse?"* (Reiter's syndrome)

I cannot stress enough the importance of asking these questions to help create your differential. You are subtly informing the examiner of your knowledge, and that you are swiftly ruling possible diagnoses in/out. You are searching for information that YOU need. You are playing the game.

Step 8   Screen for the complications of arthritic conditions, if time permits

Complications of arthritic conditions

Cardiac
- Heart block
- Pericardial effusions
- Myocardial infarctions (MI)
- Pericarditis

Haematological
- Felty's syndrome
- Pancytopenia

Neurological
- Carpal tunnel syndrome
- Cord compression secondary to atlantoaxial subluxation

Ophthalmological
- Keratoconjunctivitis sicca
- Sjögren's syndrome
- Scleritis

Respiratory
- Pulmonary fibrosis
- Rheumatoid nodules (within the pulmonary interstitium)
- Pleural effusions
- Bronchitis
- Bronchiectasis

Vasculitic
- Acute neutrophilic vasculitis
- Acute lymphocytic vasculitis

Red Flags
▶ Weight loss
▶ Resistance to analgesia
▶ Acutely red, swollen, painful joint
▶ Pain that wakes them up at night
▶ Child with a limp

Remember to ask

- Past medical history
- Past surgical history
- Drug history (they may be on potent immunosuppressants, so remember to screen for side-effects) and allergies
- Family history (arthritis or other autoimmune conditions)
- Social history (alcohol, smoking)

- *"Any loss of sensation in your legs or when you wipe your bottom?"*

Step 3   **Establish the impact this is having**

- *"What is your range of back movement like?"*

Step 4   **Build on *Step 3***

- *"Bearing that in mind, what sort of impact has this had on you and your life?"*

> **Technique alert**
>
> Back pain has a huge impact on working life! Consider this when enquiring into the impact the back pain has had.

Step 5   **Screen for any other joints that may be similarly affected**

- *"Do you have any other joints that present in a similar way?"*

Step 6   **Systemic screen**

- *"Have you lost any weight?"*
- *"Have you had a high temperature?"*
- *"Do you feel persistently tired or fatigued?"*
- *"How do you feel in general?"*

Step 7   **Create a differential**

"There are lots of things that may be responsible for causing back pain/stiffness, so I'm going to ask a few very important screening questions."

Then ask the following:
- *"Do you remember hurting your back?"* (mechanical trauma)
- *"Have you been feverish or suffered from recurrent infections?"* (infective)
- *"Is your back tender to touch?"* (infarction)
- *"Do you have any hearing loss or joint/limb deformity?"* (metabolic – Paget's disease)

You will be aware if the cause is inflammatory, i.e. rheumatoid or ankylosing spondylitis, based on the characteristics of the pain/stiffness.

Also consider whether:

- malignant – breast, thyroid, renal, myeloma, prostate, lung?
- abdominal – abdominal aortic aneurysm (AAA), pyelonephritis, ruptured ovarian cyst, peptic ulcer disease?

Remember to ask

- Past medical history
- Past surgical history
- Drug history (they may be on potent immunosuppressants, so remember to screen for side-effects) and allergies
- Family history (arthritis or other autoimmune conditions)
- Social history (alcohol, smoking)

2.3 Head trauma

Summary of steps required

1. Establish what happened
2. If there was a period of recovery, ask about deterioration
3. Establish what happened at the hospital
4. Ask about the injuries they sustained
5. Ask about any injuries they still have
6. Discuss the impact the injuries have had on them
7. Discuss rehabilitation

Step 1   Establish what happened

- *"How did your head injury happen?"* (mechanism)
- *"Specifically, did you stop quickly and over a short distance, or did you stop over a longer period of time and therefore over a longer distance (i.e. did you roll)?"*
- *"Did you lose consciousness?"* If so: *"How long were you unconscious for?"*
- *"How did you feel* immediately after *the accident?" "Was there a period of recovery, i.e. you felt fine following the incident?"*

Hint alert

- Asking about the speed and distance of stopping helps with your differential. Stopping quickly (i.e. with increased velocity) increases the risk of the patient developing a *subdural haemorrhage* and massive brain injury.
- Loss of consciousness is a good way to assess severity. Mild (6h), moderate (12h), severe (>24h).
- When asking about recovery, you are screening for a lucid interval, indicative of an *extradural haemorrhage*; i.e. if the patient feels fine immediately following the accident and subsequently starts to deteriorate some time afterwards, consider an *extradural haemorrhage*.

Step 2 **If there was a period of recovery, ask about deterioration**

- *"How long after the incident did you start to get worse?"*
- *"Did you have any nausea and vomiting?"*
- *"Did you feel drowsy and/or confused?"*
- *"Did you develop a headache?"*
- *"Did you start shaking, which led you to bite your tongue/ wet yourself?"* (screening for a seizure)
- *"Did you have any subsequent loss of consciousness?"* If so: *"How long did you lose consciousness for?"*

Hint alert

All of this information allows you to assess the type of brain injury *(primary/secondary)* and where the injury may have been sustained. This information also allows you to estimate their Glasgow Coma Score (GCS) at the time of injury; another good way to assess severity.

GCS 13	mild
GCS 9–12	moderate
GCS ≤8	severe

Step 3 **Establish what happened at the hospital**

- *"What happened when you were in hospital?"*

Step 4 **Ask about the injuries they sustained**

- *"What injuries did you sustain?"*

Very specifically, ask the following:
- *"Did you have any bruising underneath your eyes or behind your ears?"*
- *"Was there any fluid/blood from your nose/ears?"*

Hint alert

- Bruising underneath the eyes *(panda eyes)* is indicative of an *anterior cranial fossa injury.*
- Bruising behind the ears *(Battle's scar)* is indicative of a *middle cranial fossa injury.*
- Any fluid/blood from the nose *(rhinorrhoea)* is indicative of an *anterior cranial fossa injury.*
- Any fluid/blood from the ears *(otorrhoea)* is indicative of a *middle cranial fossa injury.*

Step 5   **Ask about any injuries they still have**

Specifically ask the following questions:
- *"Did you experience any:*
  - *... change in your sense of smell/taste?"* (anterior cranial fossa injury)
  - *... memory loss?"* (another way to assess severity and location of injury)
  - *... weakness or sensation loss?"* (motor cortex involved?)
  - *... seizures/hallucinations?"*
  - *... change in personality?"*
- What is their functional capability?

Step 6   **Discuss the impact the injuries have had on them**

"This whole episode must have been very traumatic and understandably very difficult; what sort of impact has this had on you?"

Information you need to establish:
- Can they work?
- How is their mood?
- What is the impact on them socially?
- If they were previously active and are now debilitated, how are they coping?
- Can they live independently?

Step 7   **Discuss rehabilitation**

It is likely they will be/have been part of a rehabilitation programme.
- *"Are you part of a rehabilitation programme?"*
- *"What is involved in this?"*
- *"Has it helped you?"*

Remember to ask
• Past medical history • Past surgical history • Drug history and allergies • Family history • Social history (alcohol, smoking)

Chapter 3

Oncology

Scenarios presented

3.1   Breast cancer 37

3.2   Haematological cancer 40

Possible scenarios to practise

Lung cancer, colorectal and additional GI malignancies are possible, but those histories are covered in their relevant sections.

3.1 Breast cancer

1. Take an adequate history of the presenting complaint: 'I found a lump'
2. Address their ICE
3. Create a differential
4. Systemic screen

Step 1 ### Take an adequate history of the presenting complaint: 'I found a lump'

Whether it is an actor or someone who has been diagnosed with cancer, the following enquiries are relevant.

- *"When did you find the lump?"*
- *"Where is the lump?"*
- *"What is the size of the lump?"*
- *"Is the lump soft/hard?"*
- *"Is it regular/irregular?"*
- *"Is it firmly attached to the breast wall or easily moveable?"*
- *"Since initially finding the lump, has it changed at all?"*

Step 2 ### Address their ICE

At this point, I think it is necessary to directly address the patient's concerns. Again, whether it is an actor or someone who has been diagnosed with cancer, the following is relevant.

- *"Finding a lump is understandably very scary, how has it made you feel?"*
- *"What are/were your concerns?"*

Technique alert

It is necessary to address their concerns here. Having an established understanding of their concerns will determine the nature of your history in terms of the tone and line of questioning. It will also allow you to use their concerns to legitimize the imposition of your own agenda – see *Step 3*.

Step 6   Address their ICE

Note that I have addressed ICE at the end for this history. Haematological malignancies present very non-specifically. It is unlikely, therefore, that your patient will come with a pre-formed idea of what they think is going on. This is very different to a patient finding a lump in the breast. Given such widespread understanding of the implications of a 'breast lump', patients are usually already thinking *'cancer'*. It is thus necessary to address their concerns earlier.

Remember to ask

- Past medical history
- Past surgical history
- Drug history and allergies:
    - are they currently undergoing/have they ever undergone chemotherapy?
    - if so, enquire into their experience, side-effects and any major complications
- Family history
- Social history

Chapter 4

Respiratory

Scenarios presented

4.1 Shortness of breath 45

4.2 Cough 51

Possible scenarios to practise

Asthma

Chronic obstructive pulmonary disease (COPD)

Lung cancer

Pulmonary embolism (PE)

Pulmonary fibrosis

4.1 Shortness of breath

This history is taken from the perspective of shortness of breath (SOB) being a new presentation.

Summary of steps required
1. Take an adequate history of the presenting complaint
2. Create a differential
3. Systemic screen
4. Enquiry into established chest pathology (if known)
5. Screen for a PE (**RED FLAGS**)
6. Screen for lung cancer

Step 1 Take an adequate history of the presenting complaint

- *"When are you short of breath?"*
- *"Are you short of breath when you lie down?"*
- *"Have you been waking up in the middle of the night gasping for air?"*
- *"What makes it worse/better?"*
- *"Can you think of any triggers?"*
- *"What time of day is it worst – early morning, at night?"*
- *"Is it seasonal?" "When it's cold?"*

Hint alert

The answers to the questions above should help build the basis of your differential.

- If the patient is short of breath when they lie down (*orthopnoea*) and wakes up in the middle of the night gasping for air (*paroxysmal nocturnal dyspnoea*), your leading differential should be an underlying cardiac cause, i.e. *heart failure.*
- If there is an obvious trigger, e.g. pollen, does the patient have *atopy* (*asthma, hay fever, eczema*)?
- Seasonal SOB is very strongly suggestive of *atopy.*
- If there is an obvious correlation with exertion, e.g. walking up stairs, establish their exercise capacity and be sure to ascertain whether it is different from their norm.

Step 2   Create a differential

Technique alert

Building a differential means you will have to ask focused and specific questions. To legitimize 'dominating' the consultation for this step, saying the following would be useful:

"So, just to swiftly summarize – you have been short of breath for the past two days, which seems to be worse in the morning and triggered by spending time in the garden. Now, there are lots of things that could be causing your breathlessness, so I'm going to ask a few very important screening questions if that's OK with you?"

Screen for additional respiratory symptoms
- Cough (any blood, sputum – yellow/green/clear)
- Chest pain – respiratory chest pain is 'pleuritic' in nature – worse upon inspiration (see *Section 5.1*)
- Wheeze

Screen for cardiac symptoms
- Any chest pain (see *Section 5.1* for cardiac-like chest pain)
- Breathlessness (covered in *Step 1*)
- Cough (pink frothy sputum)
- Dizziness
- Palpitations

- Loss of consciousness (LOC)
- Swelling of ankles and/or abdomen (oedema)

Screen for anxiety
- *"Are you short of breath in particular situations?"*
- *"Is there an associated impending sense of doom?"*
- *"Do you develop tingling in your fingers?"*

Screen for additional pancytopenic symptoms
- *"Have you been bruising/bleeding more easily?"*
- *"Have you had a fever?"*
- *"Have you suffered from recurrent infections/colds, or struggled to get over a recent cold?"*
- *"Have you been particularly tired or fatigued?"*
- *"Any recent night sweats?"*

Appropriate 'women's health' enquiry
- *"Has there been any significant change in the heaviness of your periods?"* (anaemic)
- *"Are you bloated and are you coughing up blood?"* (indicative of Meigs' syndrome)

> **Technique alert**
>
> Although this may be your respiratory station, you should exclude additional pathology. You need to demonstrate the depth of your knowledge to the examiner, and it would be unsafe in a real situation to focus on one system. By 'creating a differential', which essentially means screening for pertinent symptoms in each physiological system relevant to the presenting complaint (SOB), you're not only building a solid clinical picture, but creating a mind map of your thought process for your examiner.

Step 3   Systemic screen

- *"Have you lost any weight?"*
- *"Have you had a high temperature?"*
- *"Do you feel persistently tired or fatigued?"*
- *"How do you feel in general?"*

Step 4   Enquiry into established chest pathology (if known)

If you are aware the patient has, for example, asthma or COPD, there are specific questions you must ask.
- *"How was your asthma/COPD diagnosed?"*

- *"Does your asthma/COPD easily flare up?"* (establishing if it is brittle)
- *"Have you ever been admitted to hospital as a result of your asthma/COPD, and, if so, how frequently?"*
- *"Have you ever been admitted to an intensive care unit as a result of your asthma/COPD? Did you require intubation?"*
- *"How do you monitor your own asthma/COPD?"*

Hint alert

The three main aspects you must know when assessing the severity of someone's respiratory pathology are:

1. Whether it is brittle, i.e. easily flares up
2. Frequency of exacerbations and hospital admission
3. Medications (long-term oxygen specifically) – part of your medications enquiry later on in the history.

This will enable you to understand how severe their condition is, and the likely need for treatment/management escalation (in a real-life situation). Your examiner will be looking for you to ask these questions given the pertinence of their implication.

Step 5   Screen for a PE (see Red Flags box)

Red Flags

- ▶ Long-haul flights
- ▶ Oral contraceptive pill
- ▶ Pregnancy
- ▶ Recent cancer
- ▶ Bed-bound
- ▶ Recent surgery
- ▶ Previous clot

- *"Have you recently been abroad?"* (long-haul flights)
- *"Are you currently taking the combined oral contraceptive pill?"*
- *"Is there a chance you could be pregnant?"*
- *"Have you been diagnosed with cancer in the last 6 months?"*
- *"Have you been bed bound for the past 3 days?"*
- *"Have you had surgery in the past 4 weeks?"*
- *"Previous clot in the back of legs/lungs?"*

Hint alert

The above questions form key aspects of the **Wells score** – be sure to know the Wells score.

Step 6   Screen for lung cancer

- *"Have you had any difficulty swallowing?"*
- *"Have you developed a hoarse voice?"*
- *"Have you noticed any facial swelling?"*
- *"Have you been sweating on one side of your face?"*
- *"Have you felt any pain in the region of your hand between your thumb and index finger?"*

Hint alert

Common symptoms of pulmonary malignancy:
- Cough
- Haemoptysis
- Dyspnoea
- Chest pain
- Wheeze

To screen for local spread of pulmonary malignancy:
- Problems with swallowing are indicative of *oesophageal infiltration*.
- A hoarse voice is indicative of *recurrent laryngeal nerve palsy*.
- If they have developed facial swelling, this would indicate *superior venal cava obstruction*. If they lift their arms up above their head and subsequently develop facial swelling, this is known as *Pemberton's sign*.
- Sweating on one side of the face (anhidrosis) forms part of the triad of *Horner's syndrome*, the other two components being ptosis and miosis. This is due to invasion of the sympathetic trunk.
- Pain in the T1 dermatome suggests invasion of the brachial plexus by an apical tumour – *brachial neuritis*.

Additional complications:
- Pericarditis
- Compression of the phrenic nerve, contributing to their breathlessness due to diaphragmatic palsy
- Consider symptoms secondary to metastatic spread, e.g. bone pain
- Always remember the paraneoplastic syndromes and systemic symptoms/signs, e.g. weight loss

Remember to ask

- Past medical history:
  - hay fever?
  - eczema?
- Past surgical history
- Drug history (are they on home oxygen?) and allergies
- Family history
- Social history
  - pets
  - occupations (industrial lung disease should always be considered)
  - smoking

4.2 Cough

Summary of steps required
1. Take an adequate history of the presenting complaint
2. Create a differential
3. Systemic screen
4. Enquiry into established chest pathology (if known)
5. Screen for a PE (**RED FLAGS**)
6. Screen for lung cancer

Step 1   Take an adequate history of the presenting complaint

- *"Is your cough productive?"* (any blood, sputum – yellow/green/clear)
- *"What makes it worse/better?"*
- *"Are you aware of any triggers?"*
- *"What time of day is it worst – early morning, at night?"*
- *"Is it seasonal?" "When it's cold?"*

Step 2   Create a differential

Screen for additional respiratory symptoms
- Breathlessness
- Chest pain – respiratory chest pain is 'pleuritic' in nature – worse upon inspiration (see *Section 5.1*)
- Wheeze

Screen for cardiac symptoms
- Any chest pain (see *Section 5.1* for cardiac-like chest pain)
- Breathlessness (see *Section 4.1: SOB*)
- Cough (pink frothy sputum)
- Dizziness
- Palpitations
- Loss of consciousness
- Swelling of ankles and/or abdomen (oedema)

Screen for GORD
- *"Do you tend to cough during a meal?"*
- *"Have you been suffering from heartburn?"*

Step 3   Systemic screen

- *"Have you lost any weight?"*
- *"Have you had a high temperature?"*
- *"Do you feel persistently tired or fatigued?"*
- *"How do you feel in general?"*

Step 4   Enquiry into established chest pathology (if known)

If you are aware the patient has, for example, asthma or COPD, there are specific questions you must ask.
- *"How was your asthma/COPD diagnosed?"*
- *"Does your asthma/COPD easily flare up?"* (establishing if it is brittle)
- *"Have you ever been admitted to hospital as a result of your asthma/COPD, and, if so, how frequently?"*
- *"Have you ever been admitted to an intensive care unit as a result of your asthma/COPD? Did you require intubation?"*
- *"How do you monitor your own asthma/COPD?"*

Step 5   Screen for a PE (see **Red Flags** box)

Red Flags

- Long-haul flights
- Oral contraceptive pill
- Pregnancy
- Recent cancer
- Bed-bound
- Recent surgery
- Previous clot

- *"Have you recently been abroad?"* (long-haul flights)
- *"Are you currently taking the combined oral contraceptive pill?"*
- *"Is there a chance you could be pregnant?"*
- *"Have you been diagnosed with cancer in the last 6 months?"*
- *"Have you been bed bound for the past 3 days?"*
- *"Have you had surgery in the past 4 weeks?"*
- *"Have you had a previous clot in your lungs/the back of your legs?"*

Step 6   Screen for lung cancer

- *"Have you had any difficulties with swallowing?"*
- *"Have you developed a hoarse voice?"*
- *"Have you noticed any facial swelling?"*
- *"Have you been conscious of sweating on one side of your face?"*
- *"Have you felt any pain in the region of your hand between your thumb and index finger?"*

Remember to ask

- Past medical history:
  - hay fever?
  - eczema?
- Past surgical history
- Drug history (are they on home oxygen?) and allergies
- Family history
- Social history:
  - pets
  - occupations (industrial lung disease should always be considered)
  - smoking

Chapter 5

Cardiovascular

Scenarios presented

5.1   Chest pain (acute) 57

5.2   Chest pain (chronic) 62

5.3   Peripheral vascular disease 65

5.4   Valvular history 69

5.5   Arrhythmias 72

Possible scenarios to practise

Arrhythmias, e.g. atrial fibrillation

Cardiomyopathies

Heart failure

Myocardial infarction (MI)

Possible pacemakers

PVD

Valvular heart disease, i.e. infective endocarditis

A *"Is there anything that makes the pain better?"*

You have to ask specifics at this point:
- *"Do painkillers have an impact?"* (worrying if it is resistant to analgesia)
- *"Do you have a GTN spray?"* If yes, *"Has this made a difference?"*
- *"Have you noticed that the pain eases when you sit up?"*

T Time is an important aspect of your diagnostic work-up; see **Hint alert** box.

E *"Is there anything that makes the pain worse?"*

You have to ask specifics at this point:
- *"Have you noticed that breathing in makes the pain considerably worse?"*
- *"Have you noticed that lying down makes the pain worse, and that sitting up eases the pain?"*
- *"Have you noticed that the pain is directly correlated with exertion?"* – this leads nicely on to *Step 2*.

S Enquiry into the presence of additional symptoms will make up *Step 3*.

Hint alert

Let us run through the meaning behind some of the questions above. Bear in mind that each question has a purpose, which is essentially to provide you with the information required to build your differential.

Describe the pain
- Centrally located crushing/dull pain is very characteristic of *cardiac* pain.
- A tearing sensation is more suggestive of *aortic dissection*.
- A sharp pain is more *pleuritic* in nature, and could suggest a more *respiratory*-based pathology.

Radiation
You should know the classic radiation pattern of *'cardiac referred pain'*. The reason for this is because afferent fibres of the heart and the sensory fibres of the affected cutaneous zones enter the same spinal cord segments (T1 to T4/5) on the left side and ascend in the CNS along a common pathway.

Alleviation
- Pain that is responsive to analgesia is more suggestive of *MSK*-based pathology – this is screened for when creating your differential.

- Pain that is eased/determined by position is strongly suggestive of *pericardial* pain.
- Pain that is alleviated by GTN is strongly suggestive of *cardiac* pain.

Exacerbation
- Pain that is worsened following inspiration is very likely *pleuritic* in nature, and strongly suggestive of *respiratory*-based pathology.
- As stipulated before, pain determined by position is suggestive of *pericardial* pain.
- We will talk about the link between pain and exertion in *Step 2.*

Step 2   Exercise capacity

I cannot stress too much the importance of establishing exercise capacity. There are some very key things you need to gain from this line of questioning.
- How far can they walk before the chest pain becomes unbearable and they are forced to stop?
- Do they have the pain at rest?
- What helps them recover? (e.g. GTN spray)
- How long does it take them to recover?
- Once they have recovered, can they walk the same distance again, or does the pain occur over a shorter distance/less exertion?
- How long has this been going on for?

Hint alert

All of these questions will help you establish the severity of the situation, and whether the patient has established angina. This can help you differentiate between an acute-on-chronic presentation of chest pain and simply first presentation/acute. The patient may also have some coexisting heart failure, and the information above will allow you to establish their 'New York Heart Association (NYHA) Class':

Class 1 – No limitation on physical activity
Class 2 – Slight limitation, comfortable at rest, ordinary physical activity will cause symptomatic development
Class 3 – Marked limitation of physical activity
Class 4 – Symptoms present at rest

Step 3   Additional symptoms

Bear in mind that this is an acute presentation. *Step 4* will
cover a broader range of symptoms.

- Nausea
- Pale/grey skin
- Sweating

Step 4   Create a differential

Screen for additional cardiac symptoms

- Breathlessness
- Cough (pink frothy sputum)
- Dizziness
- Palpitations
- Loss of consciousness
- Swelling of ankles and/or abdomen (oedema)

Screen for respiratory symptoms

- Cough (any blood, sputum – yellow/green/clear)
- Breathlessness
- Wheeze

Screen for an MSK cause

- *"Have you suffered any recent chest trauma that may be
  responsible for damaging some of the muscles/bones in
  your chest?"*

Screen for a GI cause

- *"Is the pain associated with food?"*
- *"Do you develop an acid taste in your mouth* (water brash)
  when the pain comes?"

Step 5   Systemic screen

- *"Have you lost any weight?"*
- *"Have you had a high temperature?"*
- *"Do you feel persistently tired or fatigued?"*
- *"How do you feel in general?"*

Step 6   Address their ICE

Remember to ask

- Past medical history (diabetes, hypertension, high cholesterol)
- Past surgical history
- Drug history and allergies
- Family history
- Social history (smoking, alcohol)

5.2 Chest pain (chronic)

Summary of steps required

1. Take an adequate history of their MI
2. Establish what symptoms they have now and what complications they may have developed, e.g. heart failure
3. Enquire into intervention
4. Establish the impact it has had

Step 1   **Take an adequate history of their MI**

"So, I understand you have suffered from a heart attack in the past, can you tell me a little bit more about that please?"

You need to know:
- when they had it
- what symptoms they developed (brief run through SOCRATES; see inside front cover)
- whether they had established angina leading up to the actual MI – be sure to establish their exercise capacity prior to the MI.

Step 2   **Establish what symptoms they have now and what complications they may have developed, e.g. heart failure**

"So, your heart attack was approximately 20 years ago now and many people who have suffered from heart attacks can develop numerous complications, so I'm going to ask a few screening questions if that's OK?"

"What symptoms do you currently have?"
- Chest pain
- Breathlessness
- Cough (pink frothy sputum)
- Dizziness

- Palpitations
- Loss of consciousness
- Swelling of ankles and/or abdomen (oedema)

Technique alert

This is what the examiner wants. They don't want you to take a history of the MI as if the patient is presenting today with new onset chest pain; instead they want you to swiftly establish the series of events and move on to the symptoms/complications the patient has now as a result. They **will** ask you about complications. By screening for them, you've already subtly informed the examiner that you know them.

Hint alert: complications of a heart attack

Short-term
- Arrhythmias
- Left ventricular failure
- External/internal rupture
- Papillary muscle dysfunction – causing mitral valve incompetence/regurgitation
- Mural thrombosis
- Acute pericarditis

Long-term
- Chronic intractable left heart failure
- Ventricular aneurysm
- Recurrent MI
- Dressler's syndrome
- Arrhythmias

Step 3   Enquire into intervention

Hint alert

It is likely the patient will have had both surgical and medical intervention. If they have had multiple stents, be sure to ask why. There will be a reason they have failed, e.g. chronic scarring.

Step 4   Establish the impact it has had

Remember to ask
• Past medical history (diabetes, hypertension, high cholesterol)
• Past surgical history
• Drug history and allergies
• Family history
• Social history (smoking, alcohol)

5.3 Peripheral vascular disease

This history is based on a patient presenting with new 'intermittent claudication'.

Summary of steps required

1. Take an adequate history of the presenting complaint: 'intermittent claudication'
2. Ask about additional symptoms – the 6 Ps
3. Establish whether they have developed the symptoms anywhere else, e.g. hands
4. Systemic screen
5. Address ICE
6. Screen for additional cardiac symptoms
7. Screen for an AAA
8. Screen for impotence

Step 1   Take an adequate history of the presenting complaint: 'intermittent claudication'

Use SOCRATES as your starting point (see inside front cover).

S *"Where is the leg pain?"*

O *"How long has this been going on for?"*

C *"Could you describe the pain?"*

R *"Does the pain radiate?"*

A *"Is there anything that makes the pain better?"*

You have to ask specifics at this point:
- *"Do painkillers have an impact?"*
- *"Does rest make the pain better?"* If so, *"How long do you have to rest for?"*

T Time is an important aspect of your diagnostic work-up.

- *"How long is the pain there when it comes on, and how long does it take to disappear?"*

E *"Is there anything that makes the pain worse?"*

You have to ask specifics at this point:
- *"How far do you have to walk before the pain starts to develop?"*
- *"Once you have rested and the pain disappears, are you able to walk the same distance again or a reduced distance before the pain starts to recur?"*

S Enquiry into the presence of additional symptoms will make up *Step 2*.

Hint alert

All of these questions will help you establish the severity of their *PVD*. The answers to these questions will also help build your *Rutherford* and *Fontaine* (below) classification scores:

I	Asymptomatic
IIa	Mild claudication
IIb	Moderate–severe claudication
III	Ischaemic rest pain
IV	Ulceration/gangrene

Technique alert

Reporting your history back with an understanding of the severity, i.e. the classification, will earn you additional marks.

Step 2 **Ask about additional symptoms – the 6 Ps**

- Pain – already covered
- Pallor – *"Is your leg pale?"*
- Perishing coldness – *"Is your leg cold?"*
- Paraesthesia – *"Any pins and needles/loss of sensation?"*
- Paralysis – *"Any weakness?"*
- Pulseless – no need to ask

Also ask:
- *"Have you noticed any deterioration in the quality of your:*
  - *… skin?"*
  - *… nails?"*
  - *… hair?"*

Technique alert

Step 2 is vital. The 6 Ps are characteristic of an acutely ischaemic leg. Although your OSCE patient will be very stable, enquiring into the presence of the 6 Ps demonstrates to your examiner that you know exactly what to look for. You will come across as being safe and competent.

Step 3 **Establish whether they have developed these symptoms anywhere else, e.g. hands**

Step 4 **Systemic screen**

- *"Have you lost any weight?"*
- *"Have you had a high temperature?"*
- *"Do you feel persistently tired or fatigued?"*
- *"How do you feel in general?"*

Step 5 **Address ICE**

Step 6 **Screen for additional cardiac symptoms**

- Chest pain
- Breathlessness
- Cough (pink frothy sputum)
- Dizziness
- Palpitations
- Loss of consciousness
- Swelling of ankles and/or abdomen (oedema)

Step 2   Screen for rheumatic heart disease

- Joint pain
- Skin lesions/rashes
- Involuntary movements

Hint alert

These form part of your Duckett Jones' Criteria:

Major criteria
- Pancarditis (chest pain)
- Polyarthritis (joint pain)
- Erythema marginatum (skin lesions/rashes)
- Subcutaneous nodules (skin lesions/rashes)
- Chorea (involuntary movements)

Minor criteria
- Arthralgia
- Fever
- Prolonged PR interval
- Raised inflammatory markers
- Risk factors (previous rheumatic heart disease (RHD))

Step 3   Systemic screen

- *"Have you lost any weight?"*
- *"Have you had a high temperature?"*
- *"Do you feel persistently tired or fatigued?"*
- *"How do you feel in general?"*

Step 4   Screen for infective endocarditis

- *"Have you experienced any:*
  - *… swelling of the stomach?"* (splenomegaly)
  - *… problems with your waterworks?"* (risk of glomerulonephritis)
  - *… visual disturbance?"* (Roth spots)
  - *… bleeding from nails?"* (splinter haemorrhages)

Hint alert

These form part of your Duke's Criteria:

Major criteria
- Microbiological evidence – two positive blood cultures at least 12 hours apart from two separate sites
- Positive findings on an echocardiogram

Minor criteria
- Risk factors
- Fever
- Vascular phenomena, e.g. Janeway lesions
- Immunological phenomena, e.g. Osler's nodes
- Microbiological/ECHO findings not part of the major criteria

Step 5   Address ICE

Remember to ask

- Past medical history (diabetes, hypertension, high cholesterol)
- Past surgical history
- Drug history and allergies
- Family history
- Social history (smoking, alcohol)

5.5 Arrhythmias

There is nothing particularly new to cover, just follow the structure below.

Summary of steps required
1. Take an adequate history of the presenting complaint
2. Enquire into additional cardiac symptoms
3. Create a differential
4. Systemic screen
5. Address ICE

Step 1 **Take an adequate history of the presenting complaint**

Patient – *"I have recently been experiencing palpitations in my chest"*

You should ask the basics:
- *"When did this start?"*
- *"How frequently do you experience these palpitations?"*
- *"How long do they last for?"*
- *"Can you describe the sensation?"*
- *"Can you tap out the rhythm on the table?"*
- *"Can you think of any triggers?"*
- *"Is there anything that makes the palpitations better or worse?"*

Step 2 **Enquire into additional cardiac symptoms**

You – *"In addition to the palpitations in your chest, have you experienced any additional symptoms?"*

Patient may also be experiencing:
- chest pain
- breathlessness
- cough (pink frothy sputum)
- dizziness
- palpitations

- loss of consciousness
- swelling of ankles and/or abdomen (oedema)

Step 3   Create a differential

You – *"Now, there are lots of things that may be responsible for causing the symptoms you have been experiencing, so I'm going to ask some very important screening questions if that's OK with you?"*
- Respiratory symptoms (covered in *Chapter 4*)
- Anxiety symptoms (covered in *Chapter 1*)

I would recommend that the above systems form the main bulk of your differential.

Step 4   Systemic screen

Step 5   Address ICE

Chapter 6

Neurology

Scenarios presented

6.1   Headache 77

6.2   Vertigo 81

6.3   Weakness 83

6.4   Neuropathy 88

6.5   Epilepsy 90

6.6   Parkinson's disease 92

6.7   Eye 94

Possible scenarios to practise

Age-related macular degeneration

Benign paroxysmal positional vertigo (BPPV)

Fall/s

Glaucoma

Migraine

Mononeuropathies, e.g. carpal tunnel/foot drop

Motor neurone disease (MND)

Multiple sclerosis

Parkinson's

Previous stroke

Temporal arteritis

6.1 Headache

Summary of steps required

1. Take an adequate history of the presenting complaint
2. Dangerous headaches
3. Safe headaches
4. Systemic screen
5. Address ICE

Step 1   **Take an adequate history of the presenting complaint**

Use SOCRATES as your starting point (see inside front cover).

S *"Where is the pain?"*

O *"How long has this been going on for?"*

C *"Can you describe the pain?"*

R *"Does the pain move anywhere else?"*

A *"Is there anything that makes the pain better?"* (see *Steps 2* and *3* for the necessary specifics you have to ask)

T *"How long does the headache last for when it comes on, and how frequently does it occur throughout the day?"*

E *"Is there anything that makes the pain worse?"* (see *Steps 2* and *3* for the necessary specifics you have to ask)

S *"Do you have any additional symptoms apart from the pain?"* (see *Steps 2* and *3* for the necessary specifics you have to ask)

There are very important symptoms you have to screen for, but I've created separate steps for this. I strongly recommend simply asking these straightforward questions (*Step 1*) without adding too much. 'Your' enquiry will be covered in *Steps 2* and *3*. It would be useful to summarize here and gently lead into *Step 2*, as below.

"So, just to very swiftly summarize if that's OK? You have a headache very specifically located on the left side, which has been present for approximately 2–3 days. The pain is throbbing in nature and doesn't seem to radiate anywhere else. Furthermore, you have noticed that the pain is responsive to paracetamol and eases when you're in a dark room. Now, there are lots of things that may be responsible for causing a headache, so I'm going to ask a few very important screening questions if that's OK?"

Step 2   Dangerous headaches

All these are life-threatening conditions, and the questions screen for **RED FLAGS**.

Subarachnoid haemorrhage
- *"Did the headache come on very quickly?"*
- *"Did it feel like you had been hit by a baseball bat?"*
- *"Did you collapse/lose consciousness?"*

Red Flags
Collapse (subarachnoid haemorrhage)
Photophobia/rash (meningitis)
Tender temples (temporal arteritis)
Early morning vomiting (raised intracranial pressure)

Meningitis
- *"Have you found it difficult to look at light?"* (photophobia)
- *"Have you developed a rash?"*
- *"Have you developed any neck stiffness?"*

Temporal arteritis
- *"Are your temples tender to touch?"*
- *"Have you had any problems with your vision?"*
- *"Have you felt any pain in your jaw?"*
- *"Have you noticed any stiffness/weakness of your arms, particularly in the morning?"*

Temporal arteritis usually occurs in middle-aged women, and 25% will have coexisting *polymyalgia rheumatica*.

Raised intracranial pressure

- *"Is the headache considerably worse when you cough, sneeze, lean forward?"*
- *"Has there been any early morning vomiting?"*

Step 3   Safe headaches

Migraine

- *"Do you develop any warning signs such as visual disturbances/changes in smell or hearing?"*
- *"Specifically, is it a throbbing pain on one side of the head?"*
- *"When you develop the headache, do you want to walk about in the fresh open air, or hide away in a dark room and go to sleep?"*
- *"Are there any identifiable triggers?"*

> **Hint alert**
>
> Migraines are characteristically throbbing in nature, on one side of the head, and patients will usually hide themselves away in a dark room. Furthermore, patients will occasionally experience an *'aura'*, which can be visual, i.e. *complicated zigzag fortification spectra*, *scotomas,* or sensory/motor symptoms. A lot of patients will have identified a potential trigger, e.g. menstruation or the combined oral contraceptive pill.

Tension headache

- *"Is it like a tight band around your head?"*

> **Hint alert**
>
> A tension headache characteristically responds poorly to analgesia.

Medication overuse headache

- *"Have you been using any painkillers?"*
- *"If so, what, and how often?"*

> **Hint alert**
>
> Paracetamol, codeine and triptans are all worth screening for.

Cluster headache

- *"Has there been any redness of your eye?"*
- *"Have you noticed any watering of your eye, or the feeling of a stuffed nose?"*
- *"Is the pain specifically located in one of your eye sockets?"*
- *"Do you feel that you want to walk about in the open air?"*

Hint alert

Cluster headaches are six times more common in men, and can be associated with alcohol and Horner's syndrome.

Temporal neuralgia

- *"Is it like a red hot needle being poked through your eye?"*

Step 4   Systemic screen

- *"Have you lost any weight?"*
- *"Have you had a high temperature?"*
- *"Do you feel persistently tired or fatigued?"*
- *"How do you feel in general?"*

Step 5   Address ICE

Remember to ask

- Past medical history (diabetes, hypertension, high cholesterol)
- Past surgical history
- Drug history (combined oral contraceptive pill) and allergies
- Family history
- Social history (smoking, alcohol)

6.2 Vertigo

Summary of steps required

1. Take an adequate history of the presenting complaint
2. Deeper enquiry
3. Identify triggers
4. Systemic screen
5. Address ICE

Step 1 **Take an adequate history of the presenting complaint**

- *"How long has this been happening for?"*
- *"What actually happens?"*
- *"How frequently do you experience this?"*
- *"How long are the dizzy spells?"*

Step 2 **Deeper enquiry**

Any additional neurological symptoms?
- *"Have you experienced any:*
  - *... nausea and vomiting?"*
  - *... hearing loss and/or ringing in your ears?"* (tinnitus)
  - *... problems with your vision?"*
  - *... changes in sense of smell/taste?"*
  - *... swallowing problems?"*
  - *... speech problems?"*
  - *... weakness/loss of sensation anywhere?"*
  - *... loss of consciousness?"*

Any cardiac symptoms?
- *"Have you experienced any:*
  - *... palpitations?"*
  - *... chest pain?"*
  - *... breathlessness?"*

Step 3 **Identify triggers**

- *"Have you identified any triggers?"*
- *"Do you become dizzy when you turn your head, e.g. on your pillow at night?"*
- *"Do you feel dizzy when you stand up?"*

Step 4   **Systemic screen**

- *"Have you lost any weight?"*
- *"Have you had a high temperature?"*
- *"Do you feel persistently tired or fatigued?"*
- *"How do you feel in general?"*

Step 5   **Address ICE**

Hint alert: vertigo differential

- *Benign paroxysmal positional vertigo (BPPV)* – most common reason for positional vertigo. Will last for very short periods of time (up to a minute at most) and is usually triggered by head movements such as turning their head on their pillow at night.
- *Ménière's disease* – most common reason for peripheral, non-positional, intermittent vertigo. Episodes will usually last hours, and patients can have associated tinnitus and fluctuating hearing loss (the hearing loss is usually between dizzy spells).
- *Phobic vertigo* – patients may describe a feeling of distance or vagueness. This is typical of *phobic vertigo*, usually linked to anxiety.
- *Acute/chronic vestibular damage* – acute onset of vertigo that can last weeks. Usually linked with infection, e.g. *vestibular neuritis* or *labyrinthitis*, or occasionally *syphilis*, *Lyme disease* or *tuberculosis*. Patients may have a gaze-evoked nystagmus.
- *Ramsay Hunt syndrome* – due to the *herpes zoster virus*. Patients will present with vertigo, unilateral hearing loss, ipsilateral facial paresis, otalgia, herpetic vesicles and general malaise.
- *Acoustic neuroma* – unilateral hearing loss is a **RED FLAG** symptom for an acoustic neuroma. An urgent posterior cranial fossa MRI is required.

Remember to ask

- Past medical history (diabetes, hypertension, high cholesterol)
- Past surgical history
- Drug history and allergies
- Family history
- Social history (smoking, alcohol)

6.3 Weakness

The patient's weakness could be anywhere, so take an appropriate history of the presenting complaint. They could present with weakness of their face/arms/legs; just switch the focus of *Step 1*. I have made sure that you cover all necessary components in your differential screen.

Summary of steps required
1. Take an adequate history of the presenting complaint: 'weakness'
2. Screen for your 6 Ps
3. Development of symptoms elsewhere
4. Systemic screen
5. Address ICE
6. Differential screen
7. Additional review of ICE if the condition is known

Step 1   **Take an adequate history of the presenting complaint: 'weakness'**

- *"When did this weakness start?"*
- *"Was there a sudden or gradual onset of weakness?"*
- *"Do you feel perpetually weak?"*
- *"Are there periods of relapse followed by periods of recovery?"*
- *"Is there anything that makes the weakness better or worse?"*
- *"Can you think of any triggers?"*
- *"Is there an element of muscle fatigue?"*
- *"Have you noticed any changes to your muscle bulk?"*

> **Hint alert**
>
> - The speed of onset is crucial. If it was rapid with minimal warning, you should suspect a *stroke*. If the onset was gradual and prolonged, chronic neurological conditions such as *motor neurone disease* should be considered.
> - A strong element of fatigability raises suspicions for *myasthenia gravis*.
> - Periods of relapse and recovery is indicative of *multiple sclerosis*.

Step 2   Screen for your 6 Ps

Ask the patient whether, in addition to the weakness (paralysis), they have developed any of the following symptoms:
- Pain – already covered
- Pallor – *"Is your leg pale?"*
- Perishing coldness – *"Is your leg cold?"*
- Paraesthesia – *"Any pins and needles/loss of sensation?"*
- Paralysis – *"Any weakness?"*
- Pulseless – no need to ask

Also ask
- *"Have you noticed any deterioration in the quality of your:*
    - *... skin?"*
    - *... nails?"*
    - *... hair?"*

> **Technique alert**
>
> Weakness is not just a manifestation of neurological conditions. Large vessel disease such as peripheral vascular disease should be considered, which is why screening for the 6 Ps is necessary.

Step 3   Development of symptoms elsewhere

- *"Have you developed these symptoms anywhere else?"*

Step 4   Systemic screen

- *"Have you lost any weight?"*
- *"Have you had a high temperature?"*
- *"Do you feel persistently tired or fatigued?"*
- *"How do you feel in general?*

Step 5   Address ICE

Step 6   Differential screen

"There are lots of things that may be responsible for causing weakness, so I'm going to ask a few very important screening questions, if that's OK."

Create your differential by asking relevant questions for the following diagnoses.

CNS
- Space-occupying lesion (SOL)
- Head trauma
- Stroke
- Epilepsy
- Multiple sclerosis
- Meningitis
- Hypoglycaemia

Hint alert

- SOL – *"Do you have a headache that is worse when you lean forward/cough/sneeze?" "Have you had early morning vomiting?"*
- Head trauma – *"Has there been any recent trauma to your head?"*
- Stroke – screen for additional neurological symptoms: changes in vision, smell, hearing, speech, swallowing, facial weakness
- Epilepsy – *"Did you have any shaking, tongue biting, or wetting of the bed prior to the weakness?"* : could be *Todd's paresis*
- Multiple sclerosis – *"Are there periods of recovery/relapse?"*
- Meningitis – *"Have you found it painful to look at light, developed a rash or neck stiffness?"*
- Hypoglycaemia – worth screening for in acute settings

Spinal
- Any urinary symptoms?
- Any bowel symptoms?

Hint alert: spinal differential

Subacute combined degeneration of the spinal cord
This will usually present with a triad of features:
- Damage to the corticospinal tract, causing spastic paraparesis
- Peripheral neuropathy and thus loss of the ankle jerk
- Dorsal column dysfunction, causing a high stepping gait

This can be due to:
- Vitamin B12/folate deficiency
- Copper deficiency
- Cervical spondylotic myelopathy
- Hereditary spastic paraparesis
- Primary lateral sclerosis (type of MND)
- Primary progressive multiple sclerosis

Transverse myelitis
Anterior spinal artery thrombosis
Disc prolapse
Syringomyelia
Spinal shock

Neuromuscular junction
- Is there an element of fatigue?

Hint alert

Fatigue is strongly suggestive of *myasthenia gravis*.

Muscle
- Early morning stiffness/weakness?

Hint alert

This could be a muscular problem such as *dermatomyositis* or *polymyositis*.

Step 7   Additional review of ICE if the condition is known

The first review of ICE can address the patient's initial concerns about developing the weakness. If the diagnosis is known after taking your history, use *Step 7* to enquire into the impact it has had on their life as a whole, i.e. work, social, ADLs, adaptations at home, transport, mood, etc.

Remember to ask

- Past medical history (diabetes, hypertension, high cholesterol)
- Past surgical history
- Drug history and allergies
- Family history
- Social history (smoking, alcohol)

Technique alert

If the patient has had a stroke, their presentation may be a multitude of things. Take the weakness and use that as your presenting complaint (as above), and come back to the additional neurological deficit they referred to later on in your differential enquiry. This will hold your structure, and avoid unnecessary tangents and a scattergun approach.

Furthermore, if the patient presents with facial weakness, ask the relevant questions listed in *Step 1*. At *Step 2*, when you would screen for the 6 Ps if the patient presented with arm/leg weakness, ask instead about additional neurological signs such as changes in vision, smell, hearing, speech and swallowing. You can then ask about the 6 Ps as part of your differential screen.

6.4 Neuropathy

Your neuropathy history is essentially the same as your weakness history. There are just a few additions.

During *Step 1*, your enquiry into the sensation loss, be sure to ask if the patient had a bout of diarrhoea 2–3 weeks earlier. This would be suggestive of *Guillain–Barré syndrome*.

When screening for additional symptoms in *Step 2*, it may be worth screening for symptoms/signs suggestive of autonomic neuropathy associated with diabetes:
- Postural hypotension
- Impotence
- Gastric paresis
- Bladder disturbance

Step 3, an enquiry into whether they have developed the symptoms they have been discussing anywhere else, is particularly important. This information will enable you to determine the type of neuropathy:
- Mononeuropathy
- Polyneuropathy
- Mononeuritis multiplex
- Radiculopathy

Hint alert: neuropathy differential

All conditions should be screened for in *Step 5*.

Inherited:
- Charcot–Marie–Tooth disease

Inflammatory/immune
- Guillain–Barré syndrome
- Chronic idiopathic demyelinating polyneuropathy

Metabolic derangement:
- Diabetes mellitus
- Vitamin deficiencies: B12/thiamine
- Renal failure
- Liver failure
- Hyperthyroidism

Toxic and drug-induced:
- Alcohol
- Amiodarone
- Lithium
- Isoniazid
- Antibiotics
- Antipsychotics
- Vincristine

6.5 Epilepsy

Summary of steps required

1. Take an adequate history of the presenting complaint: 'seizure'
2. Address ICE
3. Systemic screen
4. Differential screen

Step 1 **Take an adequate history of the presenting complaint: 'seizure'**

- *"What actually happens/happened?"*
- *"When did you first experience an episode like this?"*
- *"How many of these episodes have you had?"*
- *"Do you get any warning signs beforehand?"* (changes in the sense of taste, smell, stomach pain, awareness/ unawareness of surroundings)
- *"What happens during the seizure?"* (how long it lasts for, ensuing behaviours, LOC)
- *"What happens afterwards?* (recognition, memory loss, sensation, symptoms)

Hint alert

- *Focal motor seizures* – jerking of the affected muscle; patients may develop a post-seizure paralysis known as *Todd's paresis*.
- *Focal sensory seizures* – unpleasant tingling *'marching'* over the body.
- *Occipital seizures* – visual features ensue, e.g. flashing lights.
- *Temporal lobe seizures* – patients will typically experience auras, i.e. unpleasant taste or smell, epigastric discomfort, déjà vu and jamais vu. The seizure itself will consist of complex and bizarre behaviour, e.g. undressing themselves and facial grimacing. There is usually a rapid recovery with amnesia of seizure events.
- *Generalized tonic–clonic* – usually described as being periods of stiffness followed by loss of consciousness and subsequent shaking.
- *Myoclonic* – early morning jerks, late childhood.
- *Absent seizures* – early childhood, likely to remit fully by adolescence.

Step 2   **Address ICE**

Step 3   **Systemic screen**

- *"Have you lost any weight?"*
- *"Have you had a high temperature?"*
- *"Do you feel persistently tired or fatigued?"*
- *"How do you feel in general?"*

Step 4   **Differential screen**

This is the same as in *Sections 6.3: Weakness* and *6.4: Neuropathy*.

Remember to ask

- Past medical history (diabetes, hypertension, high cholesterol)
- Past surgical history
- Drug history and allergies
- Family history
- Social history (smoking, alcohol)

6.7 Eye

This history is applicable to various ophthalmological presentations such as red eye, blurred vision, etc. Furthermore, be aware that eye disease can be a manifestation of many diseases, such as inflammatory bowel disease (IBD), arthritis and neurological conditions.

Summary of steps required

1. Take an adequate history of the presenting complaint
2. Establish what aspect of their vision is troubling them
3. What is the actual disturbance in their vision?
4. Deeper enquiry
5. Systemic screen
6. Address ICE

Step 1 **Take an adequate history of the presenting complaint**

Make sure you establish which eye:
- Right or left eye?
- Or both?

Step 2 **Establish what aspect of their vision is troubling them**

- Central part of vision affected?
- Or peripheral part?

Step 3 **What is the actual disturbance in their vision?**

- Blurred vision?
- Double vision?
- Bumping into things more often?
- Failure to recognize people's faces?
- Tunnel vision?

Step 4   Deeper enquiry

- *"Have you noticed any deterioration in the quality of your colour vision?"*
- *"How about any deterioration in the quality of your night vision?"*
- *"Is there any redness?"*
- *"Have you noticed any discharge?"*
- *"Does/do your eye/s feel gritty?"*
- *"Have you felt any pain?"*
- *"Have you experienced any recent trauma to the eye?"*
- *"Do you wear contact lenses?" "If so, are they soft or hard?"*

Step 5   Systemic screen

- *"Have you lost any weight?"*
- *"Have you had a high temperature?"*
- *"Do you feel persistently tired or fatigued?"*
- *"How do you feel in general?"*

Step 6   Address ICE

Remember to ask

- Past medical history (diabetes, hypertension, high cholesterol)
- Past surgical history
- Drug history and allergies
- Family history
- Social history (smoking, alcohol)

Chapter 7

Gastrointestinal

Scenarios presented

7.1	Liver	99
7.2	GI bleed	102
7.3	Abdominal pain	105
7.4	Change in bowel habit	109
7.5	Dysphagia	112

Possible scenarios to practise

Alcoholic liver disease

Cirrhosis of the liver – be sure to revise all possible causes

Non-alcoholic steatohepatitis (NASH)

> • *Peripheral oedema* and *ascites* are strong clinical signs indicative of hepatic dysfunction. This occurs due to the patient's reduced serological concentration of *albumin*, which is produced in the liver. Note: albumin is the most reliable serological marker of synthetic hepatic function.

Step 2   GI screen

"In addition to the symptoms we have already discussed, have you ever experienced:
- *… nausea and vomiting?"*
- *… swallowing difficulties?"*
- *… abdominal pain?"*
- *… change in bowel habit?"*
- *… urinary symptoms?"* (see *Section 10.1* for specific urinary symptoms)

Technique alert

This is your GI screen. This very briefly covers additional GI symptoms. It is a good screening tool to cover a broad range of possible pathological locations.

Step 3   Systemic screen

- *"Have you lost any weight?"*
- *"Have you had a high temperature?"*
- *"Do you feel persistently tired or fatigued?"*
- *"How do you feel in general?"*

Step 4   Jaundice screen

- *"Have you had any recent tattoos?"*
- *"Have you had any recent piercings?"*
- *"Have you recently been abroad?"*
- *"Have you recently had any unprotected sexual intercourse?"*
- *"Has there been any recent use of a hypodermic needle (e.g. drugs, blood transfusion)?"*
- *"Do you drink alcohol?"*

Hint alert

CAGE the patient if necessary:

- *"Do you feel like you need to **C**ut down on your alcohol intake?"*
- *"Do you get **A**ngry when people suggest you should cut down?"*
- *"Do you feel **G**uilty about the volume of alcohol you consume?"*
- *"Do you ever need an **E**ye opener?"*

Each affirmative answer gives 1 point. A score of ≥**2** is classed as severe.

Remember to ask

- Past medical history:
  - specifically ask about type 2 diabetes as non-alcoholic steatohepatitis (NASH) is a manifestation of metabolic syndrome
  - any recent infections (Gilbert's)
- Past surgical history
- Drug history and allergies
- Family history
- Social history

7.2 GI bleed

This could be haematemesis or a PR bleed; this history is applicable to both.

Summary of steps required

1. Take an adequate history of the presenting complaint
2. GI screen
3. Systemic screen

Step 1

Take an adequate history of the presenting complaint

- *"How much blood has there been?"*
- *"What is the colour of the blood?" "Is it bright red, dark, or the colour of coffee grounds?"*
- If it is blood in the stool:
  "Is it mixed in with the stool?"
  "Is it on top of the stool?"
  "Is it on the toilet paper?"
- *"What else is in the vomit/stool?"*
- *"How many times has this happened?"*
- *"Has it happened before?"*
- *"Have you noticed any fresh blood since?"*

Hint alert: GI bleed differential

- **Haematemesis** (vomiting of blood) can be bright red or have the appearance of coffee grounds (blood that has been altered).
- **Melaena** is the passage (per rectum) of black, offensive, tarry stool consisting of blood that has been digested (iron has become oxidized). Melaena is caused by upper GI pathology.

Upper:
- *Mallory–Weiss tear:* bright red blood, history of retching/ vomiting; consider recent alcohol use. One-off spontaneous episode.

- *Oesophageal varices*: consider in alcoholic patients with known liver cirrhosis/portal hypertension. Bright red blood, painless, copious amounts. Additional hepatic symptomatology will likely be present – see *Section 7.1*.
- *Oesophageal malignancy*: small quantities of thin or watery blood. Additional **RED FLAG** symptoms will likely be present, e.g. difficulty with swallowing solids over liquids, weight loss.
- *Oesophagitis*: small volumes of blood often streaking vomit.
- *Peptic ulcer disease*: ulcers present in the duodenum are eased following milk and food ingestion. Usually become painful 2–3 hours after food. Gastric ulcers will typically present with pain (dyspepsia) following food. Volume of blood can vary, usually bright red. Can occasionally present as iron-deficient anaemia.
- *Gastric malignancy*: typical dyspeptic symptoms, systemic symptoms such as weight loss, and either frank haematemesis or blood mixed with vomit.
- *Gastritis*: typical epigastric pain, small volumes of blood. Consider iatrogenic cause (see *red* box).
- *Dieulafoy lesion*: very rare. Arteriovenous malformation.

Lower: the more distal the pathology, the brighter and fresher the blood; it is usually on the surface of the stool or on the toilet paper.

- *Malignancy*: colorectal, sigmoid, rectal, anal.
- *Inflammatory bowel disease*: Crohn's disease/ulcerative colitis.
- *Diverticulitis*: always consider in elderly people, especially women, who have recently had a period of constipation.
- *Colitis*: infectious/inflammatory
- *Haemorrhoids, fissures, polyps*
- *Angiodysplasia*

Step 2   GI screen

- Nausea and vomiting?
- Swallowing difficulties?
- Abdominal pain?
- Change in bowel habit?
- Urinary symptoms?

Step 3   Systemic screen

- *"Have you lost any weight?"*
- *"Have you had a high temperature?"*
- *"Do you feel persistently tired or fatigued?"*
- *"How do you feel in general?"*

Remember to ask

- Past medical history:
  - specifically ask about hepatic disease, renal disease, cardiovascular disease, respiratory conditions, malignancy
  - this is all relevant for your Rockall and Blatchford score
- Past surgical history
- Drug history and allergies:
  - specifically ask about aspirin, NSAIDs, steroids, bisphosphonates, anticoagulants
- Family history
- Social history

7.3 Abdominal pain

Summary of steps required

1. Take an adequate history of the presenting complaint
2. GI screen
3. Enquire about their menstruation if patient is female
4. Deeper enquiry, building on *Step 3*
5. Systemic screen

Step 1 **Take an adequate history of the presenting complaint**

Use SOCRATES as your opening line of enquiry (see inside front cover).

Step 2 **GI screen**

- Nausea and vomiting?
- Swallowing difficulties?
- Change in bowel habit?
- Urinary symptoms?

Hint alert

Ensure you consider women's health causes by asking the questions below. This is frequently missed out by students. See *Chapter 8: Women's health* for an understanding of the meaning behind these questions.

Step 3 **Enquire about their menstruation if patient is female**

- *"How old were you when you had your first period?"* (menarche)
- *"Have your periods always been regular/irregular?"*
- *"How long is an average bleed?"*
- *"How long between each bleed?"*
- *"Have you had any recent bleeding between periods/after sexual intercourse?"*

- *"When you bleed, is it heavy or light?" "How many tampons/pads do you require?" "Do you have any clotting or night-time leaking?"*
- *"Has there been any change with your periods?"*

Step 4   Deeper enquiry, building on *Step 3*

- *"Have you had any pain with your periods beyond what you normally experience?"*
- *"Have you felt any pain on sexual intercourse?"* (dyspareunia)
- *"Has there been any discharge?"*
- *"How about any abdominal swelling/bloating?"*
- *"Have you been coughing up any blood?"*
- *"Is there a chance you could be pregnant?"*

Step 5   Systemic screen

- *"Have you lost any weight?"*
- *"Have you had a high temperature?"*
- *"Do did you feel persistently tired or fatigued?"*
- *"How do you feel in general?"*

Remember to ask

- Past medical history
- Specific women's health enquiry, if applicable:
    - smear? STI? Previous pregnancy? Contraception use? HPV vaccination? Sexual history?
- Past surgical history
- Drug history and allergies
- Family history
- Social history

Hint alert: abdominal pain differential

Right upper quadrant:
- *Right lower lobe pneumonia* – consider in elderly patients +/- positive chest symptoms
- *Biliary colic* – onset of pain following food ingestion, lasts for 1–3 hours, can radiate to the shoulder
- *Cholecystitis/cholangitis* – right upper quadrant pain, fever, jaundice (*Charcot's triad*)
- *Liver* – hepatic abscess, hepatitis, malignancy; see *Section 7.1: Liver history* for further liver symptomatology to be aware of

- Consider *renal* pathology, e.g. *pyelonephritis* which can radiate to the right upper quadrant

Left upper quadrant:
- *Left lower lobe pneumonia*
- *Pancreatitis* – severe pain 10/10, radiating through to the back
- Consider *renal* pathology, e.g. *pyelonephritis* which can radiate to the left upper quadrant
- *Splenic infarction*

Epigastric:
- *Peptic ulcer disease* – see *Section 7.2: GI bleed* for relevant symptoms/signs
- *Pancreatitis*
- *Gastritis*
- *GORD*
- *Malignancy – gastric/oesophageal*

Umbilical:
- *Aortic aneurysm* – pain that radiates straight through to the back, common in men; collapse and hypotension common
- *Gastroenteritis*
- Children – *intussusception, Meckel's diverticulum*
- *Diverticulitis*
- *Mesenteric ischaemia* – history of AF
- *Inflammatory bowel disease*
- *Irritable bowel syndrome*

Right iliac fossa:
- *Pyelonephritis*
- *Urinary tract infection*
- *Appendicitis*
- *Caecal carcinoma*
- *Inflammatory bowel disease*
- *Ovarian cyst/torsion*
- *Ectopic pregnancy*

Left iliac fossa:
- *Pyelonephritis*
- *Urinary tract infection*
- *Malignancy*
- *Diverticulitis* – elderly patients, especially female, with a recent history of constipation
- *Sigmoid volvulus*
- *Colitis* – ischaemia/ulcerative/infective
- *Ovarian cyst/torsion*
- *Ectopic pregnancy*

Subrapubic:
- *Pelvic appendicitis*
- *Pelvic inflammatory disease (PID)*
- *Endometriosis*
- *Ovarian cyst/torsion*
- *Ectopic pregnancy*
- *Fibroids*
- *Cystitis/urinary tract infection*
- *Pregnancy/miscarriage*

Other:
- *Diabetic ketoacidosis*
- *Hernias*
- *Radiation of testicular pain*
- *Lead poisoning*
- *Porphyria*

7.4 Change in bowel habit

Summary of steps required

1. Take an adequate history of the presenting complaint
2. GI screen
3. Systemic screen
4. Create a differential/screen for complications of IBD

Step 1   Take an adequate history of the presenting complaint

- *"How many times have you been visiting the toilet?"*
- *"What is normal for you?"*
- *"What is the stool consistency, colour and smell?"*
- *"Is there any blood? How much? What colour is it? Is it fresh blood? Is it mixed in with or on the surface of the stool? Or is it on the toilet paper?"*
- *"Is there any mucus?"*
- *"Do you ever experience urgency?"*
- *"When you have visited the toilet, do you feel like you have completely emptied?"*

Step 2   GI screen

- Nausea and vomiting?
- Swallowing difficulties?
- Abdominal pain?
- Urinary symptoms?

Step 3   Systemic screen

- *"Have you lost any weight?"*
- *"Have you had a high temperature?"*
- *"Do you feel persistently tired or fatigued?"*
- *"How do you feel in general?"*

Step 4   Create a differential/screen for complications of IBD

- Any mouth ulcers?
- Any visual disturbances?
- Any skin rashes/lesions?
- Any joint/back pain?
- Yellow jaundice?

Hint alert

Step 4 is particularly important if the demographic of your patient fits with a possible *IBD* diagnosis.

- Mouth ulcers are suggestive of *Crohn's disease*
- If the patient has *IBD*, *uveitis* is a well-known complication causing visual disturbances
- Patients with *Crohn's disease* can develop *pyoderma gangrenosum* and *erythema nodosum*
- Always consider *MSK* manifestations such as *polyarthritis*, *sacroiliitis* and *ankylosing spondylitis*
- Patients with *ulcerative colitis* can develop *primary sclerosing cholangitis*

Remember to ask

- Past medical history
- Past surgical history
- Drug history and allergies
- Family history
- Social history

Hint alert: change in bowel habit differential

Upper GI causes:
- *Cholestasis*
- *Pancreatic enzyme insufficiency*
- *Rapid gastric emptying* – diabetes, thyrotoxicosis

Small bowel:
- *Coeliac disease* – bloating, abdominal pain, muscular wastage (buttocks, trapezius); direct correlation with ingestion of gluten
- *IBS* – history of spasmodic abdominal pain, anxiety, change in bowel motions

- *Gastroenteritis*
- *Crohn's disease*
- *Malignancy*

Large bowel:

- *Colitis* – ischaemia/ulcerative/infective
- *Diverticular disease*
- *Malignancy*

Other:

- *Iatrogenic* – antibiotics, analgesia, laxatives, etc.
- *Electrolyte abnormalities*, e.g. *hypercalcaemia*
- *Rare conditions* – Zollinger–Ellison syndrome

7.5 Dysphagia

Summary of steps required

1. Take an adequate history of the presenting complaint
2. GI screen
3. Systemic screen

Step 1   **Take an adequate history of the presenting complaint**

- *"Do you have difficulty swallowing both solids and liquids?"*
- *"Did it start with a difficulty swallowing solids, which has now progressed to liquids?"*
- *"Do you find it difficult initiating the swallowing movement?"*
- *"Is swallowing painful?"*
- *"Do you experience any reflux?"*
- *"Does it feel like food is getting stuck?"*
- *"Do you feel you have bad breath?"*
- *"If you try really hard, are you able to swallow?"*
- *"Have you recently developed any shortness of breath, chest pain, cough, or a wheeze?"*

Hint alert

- Difficulty in swallowing both liquids and solids is indicative of *achalasia*.
- Difficulty in swallowing solids over liquids is indicative of *malignancy*.
- A problem with being able to initiate the swallowing movement is strongly suggestive of neurological compromise, e.g. *MND, stroke, myasthenia gravis*.
- Painful swallowing is suggestive of *oesophageal spasms*.
- If the patient has reflux, bad breath or food is getting stuck, this is suggestive of a *pharyngeal pouch* or possibly a *stricture*.
- If the patient is able to physically swallow, consider *globus hystericus*.

Step 2   GI screen

- Nausea and vomiting?
- Abdominal pain?
- Change in bowel habit?
- Urinary symptoms?

Step 3   Systemic screen

- *"Have you lost any weight?"*
- *"Have you had a high temperature?"*
- *"Do you feel persistently tired or fatigued?"*
- *"How do you feel in general?"*

Remember to ask
• Past medical history
• Past surgical history
• Drug history and allergies
• Family history
• Social history

8.1 Infertility

Step 1   **Establish how long they have been trying for a baby**

Make sure you enquire into how long it is they have been having sexual intercourse and ensure it is without the use of contraception.

Hint alert

Infertility investigations should be initiated after 12 months.

Step 2   **Enquiry into their menstruation**

- *"When did you have your first period?"* (menarche)
- *"Have your periods always been regular/irregular?"*
- *"How long is an average bleed?"*
- *"How long between bleeds?"*
- *"Any recent bleeding between periods/after sexual intercourse?"*
- *"When you bleed, is it heavy or light?" "How many tampons/pads do you require?" "Do you have any clotting or night-time leaking?"*
- *"Has there been any change with your periods?"*

Step 3   **Deeper enquiry, building on *Step 2***

- *"Have you had any pain with your periods beyond what you normally experience?"*

- *"Have you felt any pain on sexual intercourse?"* (dyspareunia)
- *"Have you noticed any discharge?"*
- Screen for polycystic ovaries (hair growth, weight gain, voice deepening)
- Screen for premature ovarian failure (dry vagina, facial flushing)

Hint alert

- If the patient presents with discharge and dyspareunia, this raises suspicion of *pelvic inflammatory disease.*
- If the patient presents with deep dyspareunia, cyclical dysmenorrhoea and irregular periods, consider *endometriosis* as your leading differential.
- If the patient has only recently stopped utilizing hormonal contraception, consider *hypothalamic amenorrhoea.*

Step 4   Systemic screen

- *"Have you lost any weight?"*
- *"Have you had a high temperature?"*
- *"Do you feel persistently tired or fatigued?"*
- *"How do you feel in general?"*

Step 5   Questions for the man

- Any major testicular injury?
- Any use of anabolic steroids?
- Any recent regime of chemotherapy?
- Post-pubertal mumps?
- STI?
- Is he able to successfully ejaculate?

Hint alert

In an OSCE situation, it is unlikely you will have the male in the room with you. Nevertheless, it is vital that you ask the woman questions about her partner. ALWAYS consider male factor infertility and show the examiner that you are doing so by asking about the topics in *Step 5*.

Step 6   **Have either conceived previously?**

This will allow you to differentiate between primary and secondary infertility and which person in the relationship may be infertile.

Step 7   **Assess the impact on the relationship of not being able to conceive**

Address their ICE.

Technique alert

The examiner will be waiting for you to address concerns. Infertility can have a huge impact on relationships. It is essential, therefore, that you enquire into the effect it has had. The patient/couple will 'need' an opportunity to voice their concerns, so be sure to give it to them.

Remember to ask

- Past medical history
- Specific women's health enquiry:
  - results of their most recent smear?
  - previous STI?
  - previous pregnancy? (ectopics?)
  - contraception use? (last use of contraception – *hypothalamic amenorrhoea*?)
  - HPV vaccination?
  - sexual history? (*PID*?)
- Past surgical history
- Drug history and allergies
- Family history
- Social history

Hint alert: infertility differential (female causes)

- **Hypothalamus:** *hypothalamic amenorrhoea* (recent stoppage of hormonal contraception)
- **Ovaries:** *polycystic ovaries, premature ovarian failure* (before the age of 40), previous tubal surgery/invasive investigations
- **Fallopian tubes:** *PID, torsion, previous ectopics*
- **Uterus:** *endometriosis*, PID
- **Cervix:** *Cervicitis, cervical stenosis*

8.2 Pregnancy

Step 1 **The three mandatory questions**

- Gestational age?
- Gravida para?
- Expected date of delivery?

Examples
- *"I have just been informed you are pregnant, many congratulations. I can imagine it's all very exciting, how are you feeling about things?"*
- *"And how far into your pregnancy are you?"* If they're due soon, you could follow that up with: *"Oh wow, not long to go. I can imagine it's all getting very exciting and possibly quite scary now…?"*
- *"Have you been pregnant before?" "Have you got any children?"*
- *"And what is the expected date of delivery?"*

Technique alert

I strongly suggest these questions be the start of your consultation. This will allow you to gain a good grasp of the situation, and, if said pleasantly, will help build patient rapport.

Step 2 **Enquiry into RED FLAG symptoms**

This is determined by the presenting complaint. The following enquiry covers Red Flags.
- Has the patient got a headache?
- Any visual disturbances?
- Any abdominal pain?

Red Flags

▶ Headache

▶ Visual disturbances

▶ Abdominal pain

▶ Swelling of ankles or abdomen

▶ Seizure

▶ Vaginal bleeding

- Any swelling of the ankles or abdomen?
- Any shaking with tongue biting/urinary incontinence? (seizure)
- Loss of consciousness?
- Any vaginal bleeding?

Hint alert

The development of a headache, visual disturbances, abdominal pain and oedema are all symptomatic manifestations of *pre-eclampsia*. Seizures and loss of consciousness are suggestive of *eclampsia*.

Any vaginal bleeding should be considered abnormal in pregnancy – consider *miscarriage, placenta praevia, placental abruption*.

Technique alert

It is likely you will get a normal pregnancy. If this is the case, do not be put off. Follow the line of questioning in *Step 2* to demonstrate to your examiner you are screening for **RED FLAGS** (*Step 2*). This shows you are safe and competent.

Step 3   **Additional mandatory pregnancy questions**

"You mentioned before that you are currently X weeks and this is your first pregnancy, and the expected date of delivery is Y. I'm just going to ask a few additional screening questions if that's OK?"

- Planned/unplanned? (if unplanned, were they using contraception?)
- Natural/assisted? (IVF, ovulation induction)
- Were the 12 and 20 week scans normal?
- All blood tests normal?
- Have any antibiotics been required?
- Have any additional immunizations been needed?
- Did patient opt for the fetal screening programme? If so, any problems identified?
- Expected mode of delivery?
- Any domestic abuse?

Hint alert

One in four pregnant women experiences domestic abuse.

Remember to ask

- Past medical history
- Specific women's health enquiry:
  - smear?
  - STI?
  - previous pregnancy? (ectopics?)
  - contraception use?
  - HPV vaccination?
  - sexual history?
- Past surgical history
- Drug history and allergies
- Family history
- Social history

8.3 PV bleed

Summary of steps required

1. Take an adequate history of the presenting complaint
2. Build your differential
3. Systemic screen
4. Assess the impact it is having

Step 1 **Take an adequate history of the presenting complaint**

Simply establish how long this has been going on for, the type of bleed, possible triggers, anything that makes it worse/better.

An adequate enquiry into their menstruation is also required.
- *"When did you have your first period?"* (menarche)
- *"Have your periods always been regular/irregular?"*
- *"How long is an average bleed?"*
- *"How long between bleeds?"*
- *"Have you had any recent bleeding between periods/after sexual intercourse?"*
- *"When you bleed, is it heavy or light?" "How many tampons/pads do you require?" "Have you had any clotting or night-time leaking?"*
- *"Have you noticed any change with your periods?"*
- *"Have you gone through the menopause?"*

Step 2 **Build your differential**

You need to enquire into additional symptoms to help do this.
- *"Have you had any pain with your periods beyond what you normally experience?"*
- *"Have you felt any pain on sexual intercourse?"* (dyspareunia)
- *"Have you noticed any discharge?"*
- *"Have you had any abdominal swelling/bloating/pain?"*

- *"Have you recently been coughing up blood?"* (haemoptysis)
- *"Have there been any changes to your waterworks?"* (see *Section 10.1: Urology* for relevant questions to ask)
- *"How about any changes in your bowel habit?"*
- *"Is there a chance you could be pregnant?"*
- Screen for thyroid symptoms (see *Section 9.1: Thyroid*)
- Screen for pancytopenia (see *Section 3.2: Haematological cancer*)

Hint alert: the differential for a PV bleed is vast

- If the patient has had a period of amenorrhoea and is now spontaneously bleeding, consider *pregnancy (ectopic, miscarriage)*.
- If the patient presents with deep dyspareunia, cyclical dysmenorrhoea and irregular periods/PV bleeding, consider *endometriosis* as your leading differential.
- It is very common for patients to have *ovulatory/anovulatory dysfunctional uterine bleeding*.
- *Meigs' syndrome* is a triad of pleural effusion (causing possible haemoptysis), ascites and an ovarian tumour (abdominal pain/swelling/bloating).
- *Fibroids* and *polyps* can cause irregular PV bleeding and abdominal pain/dragging sensation.
- If the patient has been through the menopause and is now presenting with PV bleeding, this is a **RED FLAG** symptom for *endometrial cancer*. If the patient has vague abdominal pain/bloating, consider *ovarian cancer*. *Cervical cancer* presents in younger generations with an extensive past sexual history and who are HPV positive (in the *Remember to ask* box below there are two lines of questioning that form part of the past medical history enquiry which will help rule cervical cancer in/out. These are the results of recent smear tests and HPV vaccination, as well as an enquiry into their sexual history).
- If the patient has menorrhagia and additional, irregular PV bleeding, that may be a sign of a more systemic *coagulation* problem. Consider screening for additional pancytopenic symptoms.
- If the patient is systemically unwell, consider *infection*.

Red Flags

- ▶ Weight loss
- ▶ Post-menopausal bleeding
- ▶ HPV positive
- ▶ Any bleeding in pregnancy

Step 3   Systemic screen

- *"Have you lost any weight?"*
- *"Have you had a high temperature?"*
- *"Do you feel persistently tired or fatigued?"*
- *"How do you feel in general?"*

Step 4   Assess the impact it is having

Address their ICE.

Remember to ask

- Past medical history
- Specific women's health enquiry:
  - smear?
  - STI?
  - previous pregnancy? (ectopics?)
  - contraception use? (combined oral contraceptive is protective in endometrial and ovarian cancer. Intrauterine devices/systems can cause PV bleeding)
  - HPV vaccination? (major risk factor for cervical cancer)
  - sexual history?
- Past surgical history
- Drug history and allergies
- Family history
- Social history

8.4 Pelvic pain

Summary of steps required

1. Take an adequate history of the presenting complaint
2. GI screen
3. Enquire about their menstruation
4. Deeper enquiry, building on *Step 3*
5. Systemic screen

Step 1 **Take an adequate history of the presenting complaint**

Use SOCRATES as your opening line of enquiry (see inside front cover).

Step 2 **GI screen**

- Nausea and vomiting?
- Swallowing difficulties?
- Change in bowel habit?
- Urinary symptoms?

Hint alert

Ensure you consider GI causes by asking the questions above. This shows the examiner the depth of your thinking. Just because this is a women's health station, and, by default, a relevant condition, doesn't mean you discard all possible diagnoses. That would be unsafe in real life.

Step 3 **Enquire about their menstruation**

- *"When did you have your first period?"* (menarche)
- *"Have your periods always been regular/irregular?"*
- *"How long is an average bleed?"*
- *"How long between bleeds?"*
- *"Have you had any recent bleeding between periods/after sexual intercourse?"*

- *"When you bleed, is it heavy or light?" "How many tampons/pads do you require?" "Have you had any clotting or night-time leaking?"*
- *"Has there been any change with your periods?"*

Step 4   Deeper enquiry, building on *Step 3*

- *"Have you had any pain with your periods beyond what you normally experience?"*
- *"Have you felt any pain on sexual intercourse?"* (dyspareunia)
- *"Have you noticed any discharge?"*
- *"Have you had any abdominal swelling/bloating?"*
- *"Have you been coughing up any blood?"*
- *"Is there a chance you could be pregnant?"*

Step 5   Systemic screen

- *"Have you lost any weight?"*
- *"Have you had a high temperature?"*
- *"Do you feel persistently tired or fatigued?"*
- *"How do you feel in general?"*

Remember to ask

- Past medical history
- Specific women's health enquiry:
  - smear?
  - STI?
  - previous pregnancy? (ectopics?)
  - contraception use?
  - HPV vaccination?
  - sexual history?
- Past surgical history
- Drug history and allergies
- Family history
- Social history

Remember to ask

- Past medical history
- Specific women's health enquiry if applicable:
  - smear?
  - STI?
  - previous pregnancy?
  - if the woman suffered from a post-partum haemorrhage (PPH), this predisposes her to the development of Sheehan's syndrome
  - contraception use? *(hypothalamic amenorrhoea)*
  - HPV vaccination?
  - sexual history?
- Past surgical history
- Drug history and allergies
- Family history:
  - very important to know when her mum went through the menopause
- Social history

Chapter 9

Endocrine

Scenarios presented

9.1   Thyroid 133

9.2   Diabetes 136

Possible scenarios to practise

Thyroid disease

Diabetes with complications

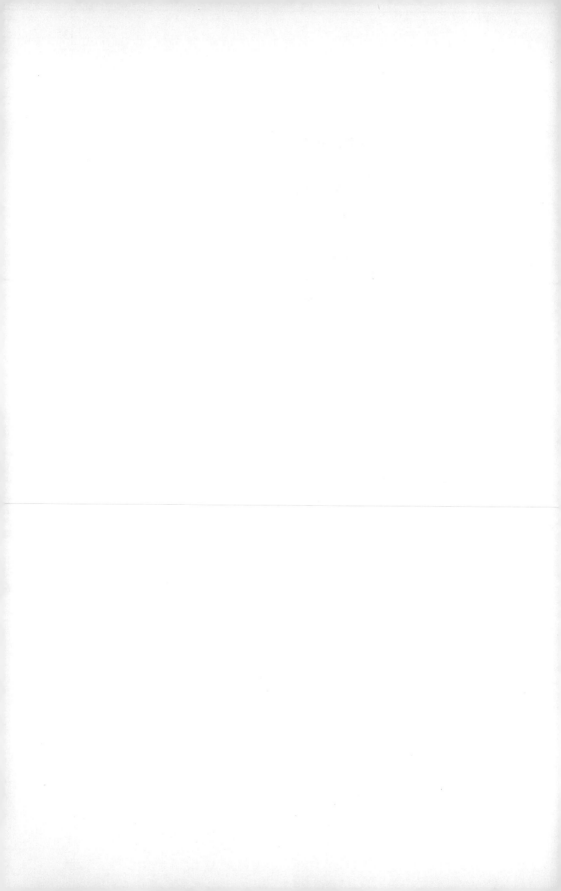

9.1 Thyroid

The presentation for thyroid disease will vary, but the following are a general set of questions that are applicable in any circumstance.

Summary of steps required
1. Take an adequate history of the presenting complaint
2. Temperature control
3. Weight control
4. Vision
5. Neck swelling
6. Early morning muscular weakness/stiffness
7. Bowel habit
8. Menstrual regularity/heaviness
9. Mood
10. Systemic screen

Step 1   Take an adequate history of the presenting complaint

- *"Have you recently been sweating a lot?"*
- *"Have you developed a tremor?"*
- *"Have you had any palpitations?"*

Step 2   Temperature control

- *"Have you noticed you have become intolerant to the heat or cold?"*

Step 3   Weight control

- *"Have you been putting on or losing weight regardless of how much you eat and/or exercise?"*

Step 4   Vision

- *"Have you developed any visual disturbances?"*

Step 5   Neck swelling

- *"Have you had any painful swelling of your neck?"*

Step 6   Early morning muscular weakness/stiffness

- *"Has there been any weakness or stiffness of your upper arms, particularly in the morning?"*

Step 7   Bowel habit

- *"Have you noticed a recent change in bowel habit?"*

Step 8   Menstrual regularity/heaviness

- *"Have you noticed a change in the regularity/heaviness of your periods?"*

Step 9   Mood

- *"Has there been any recent change in your mood?"*

Hint alert

Let us run through the meaning behind some of the questions above. In order to do this, we need to review the fundamental functions of the thyroid gland.

- Increase in *basal metabolic rate*. This contributes to temperature intolerances, i.e. heat *(hyper-)* or cold *(hypo-)*, as well as weight gain *(hypo-)* or weight loss *(hyper-)*. Furthermore, an *over-active* thyroid can cause diarrhoea and amenorrhoea; the opposite is true for an *under-active* thyroid.
- Thyroid hormones up-regulate *beta* receptors, consequently potentiating the effects of catecholamines. This has positive chronotropic and ionotropic effects on the heart, contributing to the symptomatic development of *sweating, palpitations, tremor*.
- Thyroid hormones also contribute to the development of the *nervous* and skeletal *systems*.
- Thyroid hormones stimulate protein synthesis, and increase the use of glucose and fatty acids for ATP production; they also promote lipolysis and cholesterol excretion. This contributes to weight gain/loss.
- *Goitres* (neck swellings) are characteristic of thyroid disease.
- *Exophthalmos* can contribute to disturbances in vision.
- Changes in *mood* can be secondary to thyroid disease, e.g. *anxiety* in an *over-active thyroid* and *depression* in an *under-active thyroid*.

Step 10   Systemic screen

- *"Have you lost any weight?"*
- *"Have you had a high temperature?"*
- *"Do you feel persistently tired or fatigued?"*
- *"How do you feel in general?"*

Technique alert

Thyroid symptoms are characteristically non-specific. Be sure to consider alternative diagnoses, such as *mental health* conditions. Refer to *Chapter 1: Psychiatry* for relevant mental health screening questions.

Remember to ask

- Past medical history
- Past surgical history
- Drug history and allergies
- Family history
- Social history

Hint alert: causes for hyper-/hypothyroidism

Hyperthyroidism:
- Graves' disease
- Toxic multinodular goitre
- Toxic adenoma
- Thyroiditis (de Quervain's/Hashimoto's)
- Iatrogenic (amiodarone)

Hypothyroidism:
- Graves' disease
- Autoimmune (Hashimoto's)
- Iatrogenic (treatment for hyperthyroidism, e.g. surgical ablation)
- Severe iodine deficiency (endemic)

9.2 Diabetes

The examiner will likely say the following:

"This patient has an established diagnosis of diabetes; I would like you to focus on ..."

It is important you take a history of this, and broaden your history later on with general screening questions to cover all other diabetic complications.

In my personal experiences with diabetic cases in professional exams, I have usually got an amputee. They had usually developed PVD with superimposed diabetic neuropathy. The *Step 1* aspect of my history was a PVD history (refer to *Chapter 5: Cardiovascular*). I then asked about the intervention they have had for that particular problem (usually surgical).

I then stated:

"So, I understand how your diabetes presented, and also the management you have had for that particular complication. Before I move on to the remainder of my history, given how systemic diabetes can be, I am going to ask a few screening questions if that's OK? I'd just like to establish how advanced your diabetes is."

This structure to your history can be used regardless of the diabetic presentation. Just switch the focus of your *Step 1* enquiry according to their presenting complaint.

The following history is based on the presenting complaint being intermittent claudication, i.e. the patient has developed PVD secondary to their diabetes.

Summary of steps required

1. Take an adequate history of the presenting complaint: 'intermittent claudication'
2. Ask about additional symptoms – the 6 Ps
3. Establish whether they have developed these symptoms anywhere else, e.g. hands
4. Systemic screen
5. Address ICE
6. Address the management for that particular complication (expect an amputee)
7. Screen for all other complications
8. Address overall diabetic management

Step 1   **Take an adequate history of the initial presenting complaint: 'intermittent claudication'**

Use SOCRATES as your starting point (see inside front cover).

S *"Where is the leg pain?"*

O *"How long has this been going on for?"*

C *"Could you describe the pain?"*

R *"Does the pain radiate?"*

A *"Is there anything that makes the pain better?"*

You have to ask specifics at this point:
- *"Do painkillers have an impact?"*
- *"Does rest make the pain better?" "How long do you have to rest for?"*

T Time is an important aspect of your diagnostic work-up.

- *"How long is the pain there when it comes on, and how long does it take to disappear?"*

E *"Is there anything that makes the pain worse?"*

You have to ask specifics at this point:
- *"How far do you have to walk before the pain starts to develop?"*
- *"Once you have rested and the pain disappears, are you able to walk the same distance again or a reduced distance before the pain starts to recur?"*

S Enquiry into the presence of additional symptoms will make up *Step 2*.

Step 2   Ask about additional symptoms – the 6 Ps

- Pain – already covered
- Pallor – *"Was your leg pale?"*
- Perishing coldness – *"Was your leg cold?"*
- Paraesthesia – *"Any pins and needles/loss of sensation?"*
- Paralysis – *"Any weakness?"*
- Pulseless – no need to ask

Also ask:

- *"Have you noticed any deterioration in the quality of your:*
  - *… skin?"*
  - *… nails?"*
  - *… hair?"*

Step 3   Establish whether they have developed these symptoms anywhere else, e.g. hands

Step 4   Systemic screen

- *"Had you lost any weight?"*
- *"Had you had a high temperature?"*
- *"Did you feel persistently tired or fatigued?"*
- *"How do you feel in general?"*

Step 5   Address ICE

Step 6   Address the management for that particular complication (expect an amputee)

- *"So, I understand you have well-established diabetes, which is responsible for causing what we have been discussing. Before I move on, what management have you had for this specific complication?"*

> **Technique alert**
>
> Expect an amputee or some form of surgical intervention. Establishing exactly what happened for this whole episode is good for completeness. You can then signpost this and move on to the broader complications of diabetes – see *Step 7*.

Step 7   Screen for all other complications

- *"So, I understand how your diabetes presented, and also the management you have had for that particular complication. Before I move on to the remainder of my history, given how systemic diabetes can be, I am going to ask a few screening questions if that's OK? Just to establish how advanced your diabetes is."*

Hint alert: complications

Microvascular

Eyes: ask if there are any problems. If there are, is it because they developed symptoms or was it picked up on screening? How often do they have an ophthalmology review?

Kidneys: same enquiry! How often do they have a renal review?

Neuropathy: same enquiry! If they have diabetic feet, how often are they seen by a podiatrist? Any changes to their footwear?

Macrovascular

Screen for large vessel disease. Any *strokes/MIs*? *PVD*? Again, picked up on screening or due to the development of symptoms?

Step 8   Address overall diabetic management

- What medications do they take?
- Any side-effects?
- Have they ever required hospital admission?

Remember to ask

- Past medical history:
  - remember to enquire into conditions such as hypertension, high cholesterol, etc.; you MAY be asked about their cardiovascular risk
- Past surgical history
- Drug history and allergies
- Family history
- Social history

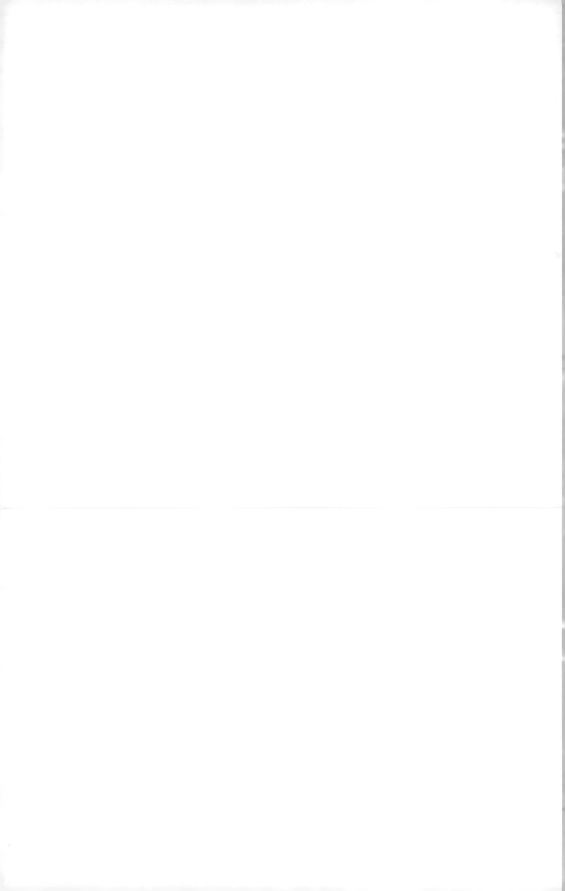

10.1 Urology

This history is applicable to various urological presentations, e.g. dysuria or haematuria. The general screening questions (*Step 1*) cover the basis of your major differential diagnoses.

Summary of steps required

1. General screening questions
2. GI screen
3. **RED FLAG** screen
4. Systemic screen

Step 1 **General screening questions**

- *"Have you noticed a change in the smell of your wee?"*
- *"Have you noticed a change in the colour?"*
- *"Is there any blood in your wee?"* (haematuria)
- *"Is it painful when you wee?"* (dysuria)
- *"Have you noticed any dribbling, specifically at the end of your stream?"* (terminal dribbling)
- *"Do you struggle to start the stream?"* (hesitancy)
- *"Has there been an increase in frequency?"*
- *"Have you been going more frequently at night?"* (nocturia)
- *"Do you ever get a sudden urge to go for a wee, and you simply cannot hold it in?"* (urgency)
- *"Do you feel like you have fully emptied?"*

Hint alert

Let us run through the meaning behind some of the questions above. Bear in mind that each question has a purpose, which is to essentially provide you with the information required to build your differential.

- *Dysuria* is one of the clinical symptoms that form a triad of legitimate clinical evidence for a *urinary tract infection (UTI)*, the other two being abdominal pain *(suprapubic)* and increased *frequency*.

- *Hesitancy* and *terminal dribbling* are **RED FLAG** symptoms, indicative of possible *prostate cancer* or *benign prostatic hypertrophy (BPH)*. An International Prostate Symptom Score (IPSS) questionnaire is a useful way to explore this further.
- If you are concerned about a possible *sexually transmitted infection (STI)*, discharge is an additional important query.
- *Haematuria* has lots of differentials. Attribute the following to key components of the urinary tract (renal pelvis, pelvi-ureteric junction, ureter, vesico-ureteric junction, bladder, urethra): trauma, tumour, infection, inflammation, stone.

Step 2   GI screen

- Nausea and vomiting?
- Swallowing difficulties?
- Abdominal pain?
- Change in bowel habit?

Step 3   **Red Flag** screen

- *"Have you had any joint or back pain?"*
- *"Have you felt any weakness or loss of sensation in your legs?"*

Hint alert

If *prostate cancer* is one of your differentials, it will commonly metastasize to the back, causing considerable back pain and possible *malignant spinal cord compression*.

Step 4   Systemic screen

- *"Have you lost any weight?"*
- *"Have you had a high temperature?"*
- *"Do you feel persistently tired or fatigued?"*
- *"How do you feel in general?"*

Red Flags

▶ Joint or back pain

▶ Weakness or loss of sensation in legs

Remember to ask

- Past medical history
- Past surgical history
- Drug history and allergies
- Family history
- Social history

10.2 Renal history

This history depends on how the patient is presenting. It is likely they will have either had a transplant or are currently undergoing dialysis. The following steps are the order in which you should structure your history.

Summary of steps required for a transplant patient

1. Brief review of diagnosis (how they presented and what ultimately led/caused them to develop renal disease)
2. Ask about the transplant
3. Ask about the symptoms now and complications
4. Ask about other intervention; they will have likely have had dialysis

Summary of steps required for a dialysis patient

1. Brief review of diagnosis (how they presented and what ultimately led/caused them to develop renal disease)
2. Ask about the dialysis
3. Ask about the symptoms now and complications
4. Ask about other intervention

Technique alert

The structure to the above histories is similar to that of your 'previous MI' history (*Section 5.2*). The examiner doesn't want you to take a history as if the patient is presenting for the first time, they want you to swiftly accrue an understanding of what happened (i.e. how they presented and what ultimately led/caused them to develop CKD), and then move on to their present situation. If the patient has had a transplant or is currently undergoing dialysis, ask about it (*Step* 2). Be sure to enquire into ICE. Then move on to *Step 3*. Establish what is happening right now, e.g. symptoms secondary to their well-established CKD, or maybe the dialysis/transplant. Symptoms that may be worth screening for are given below; by asking such questions you are subtly informing the examiner of your breadth of knowledge.

Symptoms to screen for

Urinary symptoms – kidneys are responsible for the regulation of blood volume and osmolarity, as well as the elimination of waste products (filtration).

- *"Have you noticed a change in the smell of your wee?"*
- *"Have you noticed a change in the colour?"*
- *"Has there been any blood in your wee?"* (haematuria)
- *"Is it painful?"* (dysuria)
- *"Have you noticed any dribbling, specifically at the end of your stream?"* (terminal dribbling)
- *"Do you struggle to start the stream?"* (hesitancy)
- *"Has there been an increase in frequency?"*
- *"Have you been going more frequently at night?"* (nocturia)
- *"Do you ever get a sudden urge to go for a wee, and you simply cannot hold it in?"* (urgency)
- *"Do you feel like you have fully emptied?"*

The retention of fluid – due to defunct filtration capability.

- *"Have you had any swelling of your ankles?"* (peripheral oedema)
- *"How about any swelling of your tummy?"* (ascites)

Screen for uraemic symptoms – kidneys are responsible for the elimination of waste products.

- *"Have you had any nausea and vomiting?"*
- *"Have you felt drowsy and/or confused?"*
- *"Did you develop a headache?"*
- *"Did you have any shaking episodes and bite your tongue?"* (seizure)
- *"Did you lose consciousness?"*

Screening for things like hyperkalaemia – kidneys are responsible for the serological concentration of various ions.

- *"Have you ever had an emergency admission to hospital requiring emergency treatment/dialysis?"*

Hyperphosphataemia and VWF problems.

- *"Have you noticed you bruise more easily?"*
- *"Have you noticed you itch more?"*

Renal bone disease – vitamin D metabolism.

- *"Have you developed any joint/back pain?"*

Systemic screen – kidneys pump out erythropoietin so the patient may be tired due to anaemia.

- *"Have you been feeling breathless?"*
- *"Have you recently been tired or fatigued?"*

Hint alert

Kidneys also contribute to the regulation of:

- blood pressure
- blood PH
- glucose metabolism

Immediate indications for dialysis

- Pulmonary oedema
- Potassium >6.5
- Acidotic <7.2
- Pericarditis
- Encephalopathy

10.3 Example renal consultation

Examiner – *"This patient has had a renal transplant. I would like you to talk to them about this."*

Step 1   Brief review of diagnosis

We will start as if the introductory phase is over (names, etc.).

"So, I've just been told that you have established kidney disease and you have had a transplant. Could you tell me a little bit more about that, please?"

Hopefully, the patient will provide you with some basic information, such as when they developed the renal disease, what symptoms they started to experience, etc.

If the patient does not volunteer the information you need, simply ask. And be sure to screen for some of the symptoms they may have been experiencing. Keep this brief; remember the examiner doesn't want you to take a history as if this is the patient's first presentation.

Step 2   Ask about the transplant

"So, I understand what symptoms you started to experience when you were initially diagnosed with kidney disease, and also how you were diagnosed. Ultimately, you have had a transplant. Could you talk to me about why the transplant was necessary and your experience, please?"

Hopefully the patient will volunteer the information you want, such as when they had the transplant, why it was necessary, some donor information, etc.

Step 3   Symptoms they experience now

Use this as an opportunity to summarize, then review what symptoms they have now. Furthermore, they may experience symptoms due to the medication they're taking.

Step 4   Ask about other intervention

"We have talked about your diagnosis, transplant, and indeed the symptoms you currently experience. What other intervention have you had for your kidney disease?" Dialysis is likely.

Remember to ask

- Past medical history
- Past surgical history
- Drug history and allergies:
  - the patient will likely be on immunosuppressant medication. They may have developed many side-effects; be sure to ask.
- Family history
- Social history

Assess the following when acquiring key aspects of the presenting complaint:

- When it started
- Rapid onset or gradual development of symptoms
- How long the symptoms have been present
- Anything that makes the symptoms better/worse

Step 2   Ask about additional SYMPTOMS

General: behaviour, engagement (e.g. level of playing activity in comparison to their norm), level of hunger, fever, growth, weight, rashes, dehydration

Cardio/resp.: noisy breathing (stridor, wheeze), cough, dyspnoea, cyanosis

GI: abdominal pain (colic, drawing knees up to stomach), diarrhoea, constipation, vomiting

Neuromuscular: convulsions, tongue biting, incontinence, hypotonic, abnormal movements (e.g. jerks), headaches, turning away from light

ENT: sore throat, earache, noisy breathing (snoring)

Genitourinary: screen for urinary symptoms, any nappy wetting, bed wetting

This is a bit like your 'systemic screen' in previous sections. One of my 'pet hates', as I've stated before, is taking a generic history from each system. I think this lacks clinical acumen and wastes time. However, bear in mind that the information an adult patient may volunteer will not necessarily be readily available in a paediatric case. Indeed, parents will usually be of considerable help, and depending on the child's age you may have to solely take a history from the parent. Nevertheless, to be safe, I strongly advise that you screen for concerning symptoms in each system (see *Hint alert* box above). This demonstrates to your examiner that you are being safe and will help build your differential from an otherwise vague and unhelpful history.

Mandatory section

Having established the reason the child has been brought in to see you (*Steps 1* and *2*), you now have to ask what I consider to be mandatory paediatric questions. This is an enquiry that enables you to gauge the child's overall health and wellbeing.

Step 3   Birth

Pregnancy
- Natural/assisted?
- Were the 12 and 20 week scans normal?
- All blood tests normal?
- Were any additional immunizations/antibiotics required?
- Maternal illness/drug abuse?

Birth history
- Gestational age?
- Mode of delivery?
- Any neonatal problems? Did the newborn pass meconium within the first 24 hours, require any supplemental oxygen or resuscitation, experience any birth injury or feeding problems; were they born with an infection or jaundice?

Step 4   Feeding

- Breastfed? (how long?)
- Bottlefed? (how long? which formula?)
- Weaning time?
- Transition to fully solid diet?

Step 5   Growth

- Weight/s – they may have their Red Book
- Puberty age?

Step 6   Development

- Any concerns?
- School progress?

Developmental screen <5 years
- Smiling by 6 weeks
- Sitting by 9 months
- Turns to sounds by 6 months
- First words by 18 months

- Walking by 18 months
- Talking three-word sentences by 3 years

Step 7   **Additional important questions**

- *"Is your child up to date with all their vaccinations?"*
- *"Have they been admitted to hospital for any reason other than what we have been discussing?"*
- Screen home life accordingly – if the child has asthma, does anyone smoke at home?

Remember to ask
• Past medical history • Past surgical history • Drug history and allergies • Family history • Social history